START *Dancin'* and *Don't Stop*

START DANCIN' AND DON'T STOP!

Published by Chaplain Publishing

3104 County Road 7520
Lubbock, TX 79423
www.chaplainpublishing.com

Copyright © 2015 by Kate Asbill.

Library of Congress Control Number: 2015950721

ISBN: 978-1-941549-08-7

Cover image titled Bailando by Candy Mayer
www.candymayer.com

Cover and text design: NiTROhype Creative

www.nitrohype.com

Printed in the United States of America

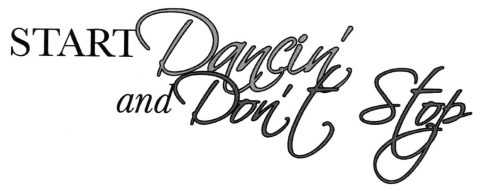

START Dancin' and Don't Stop

Thrive, Don't Just Survive!

Dr. Kate Null Asbill

Kate Null Asbill, Ed.D

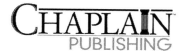

CHAPLAIN PUBLISHING

Dedication

This book is dedicated to Essie Phillips and Mary Jane Cottingham, my "Dancing Queens," with appreciation for their inspiration and their example.

It is written with much love and gratitude in memory of my mother and daddy, Dollie and John Null, and my grandmother, Maw—Ovie Parker Lueders Blankenburg.

I thank each of the precious people who have helped me to learn about life and who have taught me much through their examples of lives well lived.

I thank my brother Ronnie Null for his assistance with editing and for his encouragement through the process of writing this book.

I thank my husband, Vernon Asbill, for his steadfast love and for being my partner in this wonderful dance of life.

12-3-15

Dear Jack,

Thank you for helping me become a best selling author!

Keep on Dancin'!

Sincerely,

Kate

Contents

Introduction

"There are a lot of myths about old age," she offered.

"Like what?" I asked, curious to hear all that she had to say.

"Like you can't have sex; you can."

I thought, *That will be good news to a lot of folks.*

I was sitting in the beauty school with my feet in soapy water when I met her. She was next to me with curler rods and cotton in her hair.

"I always do my own toes," she told me. "You have to be quite a contortionist to do that."

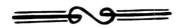

"I won this pedicure at the Ducky Affair Fundraiser," I said, feeling lucky and blessed. As we continued our conversation, I quickly realized that the real blessing of the day was meeting Virginia.

In thirty minutes she summed up almost everything my years of research had revealed. After visiting with Virginia, it came clear to me that I finally needed to begin writing my long-awaited book.

As she told me about herself, she didn't know I was taking mental notes on every word she shared. The beauty school intern doing my toes asked her, "How old are you?"

Apparently the young woman had yet to learn the lessons of Tact 101. Nevertheless, I was glad she asked and that Virginia answered, "85."

"Wow. That's the same age my Mama would be if she were still here.

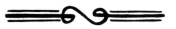

I'm writing a book called *Start Dancin' and Don't Stop*, and I'd like to hear what you have to say about what we can do to live better longer."

"I live out in Happy Valley, and I have cats and dogs and chickens. I moved here four years ago, and I immediately got involved with Senior Olympics, and I've won a lot of medals. I bowl, I golf, and I play pool."

As she talked on, I learned that she worked in labs all her life—starting when she was 15. She raised four daughters who have successful careers, and she has many interests.

"You have to keep your mind busy," she advised. "I read a lot. I love to read. I play bridge. I grew up in Canada, and my mother taught all of us kids to play games. It doesn't matter what you do—you just have to stay active."

I was going through a mental

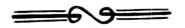

checklist of things I had concluded are vital for longevity, and she touched on almost all of them.

Each bit of advice she shared reminded me of someone I had interviewed or studied for my pro-active aging project. I knew it was time to record those revelations and pass them on—time to share what I had learned from admired elders.

Her comment about sex reminded me of a man named Maverick, who my brother Ronnie met on Bright Angel Trail as he hiked down to the bottom of Grand Canyon.

Maverick was visiting with everyone along the trail as he hiked the steep incline on the way out. He proudly bragged that he was 82 years old and that he had hiked the canyon rim to rim 100 times the year before.

Ronnie said, "My sister is doing research on aging. She will want to

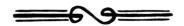

know your secret. If you don't mind my asking, "What is it?"

Without hesitation, Maverick said, "Sex, four times a week! There may be snow on the roof, but there's still fire in the fireplace!"

My brother was anxious to tell me that he had learned a secret of the universe. We were impressed to hear about Maverick's accomplishments—his stamina on Bright Angel Trail and his bedroom prowess.

Maverick's philosophy about the fountain of youth is only one of many interesting ideas I have heard. I am excited to tell you about what I have learned from all the people I interviewed from 78 to 108 about pro-active aging. I am happy to share this information and trust that it will be beneficial to you, the reader.

Hopefully, *Start Dancin' and Don't Stop* will inspire you to be more

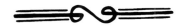

mindful about daily decisions, more positive about the aging process, and more intentional about joyfully living life to the fullest.

It is my prayer that you will thrive and not just survive!

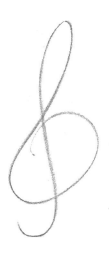

GuiDANCE:

Do you have any negative perceptions about aging that need to be examined?

What interesting characters have you met along the trail of life?

chapter *1*

Intentionally Invite Yourself to Live Better Longer

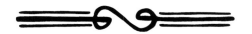

Essie, age 92, hopped out of my car and quickly hurried up the handicapped ramp on her way to vote. She carried her cane, but she hardly used it. I had the feeling she carried it in case she wanted to whack someone. She would often park it somewhere and walk off without it—forgetting

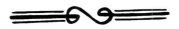

her need for the balance provided by the walking stick. After observing my dear friend and analyzing her actions, I said, "Essie, you did something right. What did you do to be in such good shape at 92? Did you exercise?"

"Oh, yeah," she said, smiling as she remembered. "Me and Mary Jane used to go line dancing over at San Jose Senior Center—and when we finished there, we went to Northgate and danced some more!"

My passing observations of Essie's ability to maneuver easily at an advanced age prompted me to go on a quest to discern the secrets of proactive aging. I began to think about aging with intention and how, perhaps, we can age less.

Since that conversation with precious little Essie, I've given a lot of thought to the aging process, and I am certain that we have a choice of

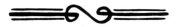

how we are going to age. After interviewing and observing many admired
elders, I am convinced that the daily
decisions we make throughout our
lives can determine both the quality
and length of our days on earth.

Much has been written about
aging, and my on-going research on
the subject confirms my belief that
there are things we can do to live better longer—to live well.

Aging is a timely topic that is of
interest to baby boomers and those
below and beyond that age group. As
one doctor told me, "The information
is out there; the research is in. People
just have to follow it." We all know
what to do. The challenge is to get
ourselves to do it. My purpose in writing this book is to distill some of that
ocean of information into doable daily
actions.

My interest in pro-active aging ac-

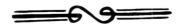

tually began many years ago when I was in high school. After visiting with my grumpy, sad-faced grandpa, I told Mama, "I'm going to sleep smiling so that when I get old I'll have an up mouth." For a while I was intentional about going to sleep with a smile on my face. I've never forgotten that decision to cultivate a cheerful countenance and now, at 60+, at least I have "happy wrinkles."

It was twenty years later before I discovered the secret of *intentionality*, but it is a subject that has impacted my life since 1985. At that time I met Dr. William Purkey and embraced his philosophy of Invitational Education. That summer I attended my first conference of the Alliance for Invitational Education, and I soon came to the realization that the IE encompassed much more than education. I thought, *What they are really talking about is intentional invitational liv-*

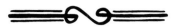

ing. It is not something you turn on and off at the schoolhouse door. It is a way of life, a way of being, a way of relating to everyone you meet. I felt as if I had plugged into the mainstream of people who thought as I did about inviting school success, about how schools should be, and most importantly, about how to live.

I became active in the Alliance for Invitational Education and began to share that philosophy with anyone who would listen. I purposefully applied the concepts to my personal life as well.

In the book, *Inviting School Success*, by Dr. William Purkey and Dr. John Novak, the authors outline the tenets of Invitational Education. The basic stance is one of trust, respect, optimism, and intentionality.[1] Although I had not heard the word intentionality before 1985, it soon became a guiding force in my life—

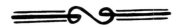

both personally and professionally.

Intentionality is the process of making a conscious choice to behave in a certain manner. Dr. Purkey says that is it about **"life being aware of itself."** When we give conscious thought to our actions and to the possible consequences of our actions, we can make better decisions. When we become aware of how we want our lives to be, we can make better choices.

Before Grandpa suffered a debilitating stroke that left him unable to speak, he once said, "If I'd have known I was gonna live this damn long I would have taken better care of myself." We have probably all heard someone make a similar statement. The reason is because of the truth it contains. If we choose to take better care of ourselves, we significantly increase our chances of *living better longer*. We do have a choice in the

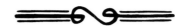

matter. We can intentionally invite ourselves to live better longer and to age less—to thrive and not just survive!

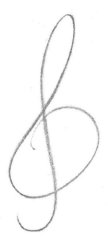

GuiDANCE:

What intentional actions will you choose today to better care for yourself?

chapter 2

Start Dancin' and Don't Stop

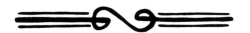

Lively little Essie inspired me to join line dancing at the Senior Citizen Center. It is great exercise, the fellowship is fabulous, and it's fun! It has been part of my weekly schedule for ten years now, and I am reaping the benefits of dancing regularly.

I have met some wonderful women

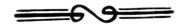

there, and I'll never forget the day I met Mary Jane.

We were standing in the hall during the break, and I asked her name. She told me and then asked mine.

I told her, "Kate Asbill."

She said, "Oh! My friend Essie used to talk about you!"

I quickly replied, "What did you say your name was?"

"Mary Jane."

I was so excited! "Oh my gosh! It's YOU!" I exclaimed. "Essie told me how you used to go line dancing together, and you're still here!!" Essie had been dead for about a year at that point.

Mary Jane and I quickly became friends, and I was happy every time I saw her stroll into the senior center.

She may have been late, but she was still there! Still dancing! She had

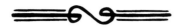

rhythm, and she was smooth on her feet. If she didn't know the steps, she just kept moving to the music. I believe there is a lot to be said for **showing up**! But, Mary Jane didn't just show up. She always had a good time, and she was an excellent example for me and for anyone else who was paying attention.

Mary Jane didn't discuss age. She said, "Age is just a number, and mine is unlisted!"

I told her, "I've heard that age is 'mind over matter.' If you don't mind, it doesn't matter."

When she passed away, several of us were curious to see if her age would be listed in her obituary. It was. We finally found out that our little "line-dancing queen" lived to be 98 years of age. By our calculations, she still showed up and danced regularly until she was 97! What a woman!

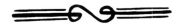

I decided to dedicate this book to my dear dancing friends, Essie and Mary Jane. The idea for the title came from a conversation with another favorite friend, Reid. He told me that one of his older friends had passed away. He said, "I wish you could have interviewed her."

I asked, "What do you think she would have told me?"

He smiled and said, "Start dancin' and don't stop!" I think Essie and Mary Jane would agree.

I know my friend Clayton would too.

I met Clayton in a honky-tonk in Texas. It was New Year's Eve and I went to the Broken Spoke in Austin with my Uncle Bobby and Aunt Maureen. Vernon was deer hunting with our grandson, Addison, so I had no dance partner. Uncle Bobby knew about my interest in older folks and also that I like to two-step. Bobby spotted Clayton when he walked in and signaled for him to come over to our table. He introduced us, and I could tell it was going to be a memorable New Year's Eve.

Clayton was 92 at that time, and he was quite a character. With a sparkle in his eye, he told me that he had a girlfriend and then added, "She doesn't like to dance, but she doesn't care if I do." I danced with him several times that evening, and I took pictures of him dancing because I knew instantly that he was my new hero. He had fun posing for the photos. He danced all night long—looking for lovely ladies without a partner and providing entertainment for everyone at the Broken Spoke.

About a year and a half later, I saw Clayton again. Vernon and I went to the South Austin Senior Center where Uncle Bobby and his band were

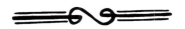

playing. He had assembled a group of experienced musicians, and they had recently released a CD called *Still Swinging in Texas*. As they played all the popular oldies, the dance floor was filled with senior citizens having fun—still swinging. Clayton was doing his best to make sure no one felt like a wallflower. There was a line of ladies who were waiting to dance, and Clayton was doing what he could to keep them happy. He would take them out, one by one, for a spin around the dance floor. Although I had a partner that night, I did get to dance with Clayton and learn a little more about him. I couldn't keep him long though because the ladies were waiting. His girlfriend didn't know what she was missing.

There's a country music song that Lee Ann Womack sings that says it this way: "And if you get the choice to sit it out or dance, I hope you'll dance."

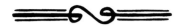

I hope you'll dance. Be like Essie, Mary Jane, and Clayton—start dancin' and don't stop!

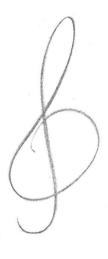

GuiDANCE:

Are you sittin' it out or are you dancin'?

chapter 3

Live Fast, Love Hard, Die Young, and Leave a Beautiful Memory

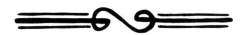

When I first told my brother Ronnie I was writing a book about how we can live better longer, he said, "I don't want to live to be 100. I think you should have a chapter called 'Live Fast, Love Hard, Die Young, and Leave a Beautiful Memory.'" He's not the only one to express that sentiment.

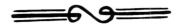

As I have talked to people about my research on aging, many have said, "I don't want to live a long time." That's why the first chapter of the book is called "Intentionally Invite Yourself to Live Better Longer." It doesn't say how long that might be.

One trusted advisor recommended, "You need a number in your book title." But there are a myriad of books and articles about "How to Live to be 100" and, although it sounds like a good idea to me, others don't see it that way. I even saw one article about living to be 150, but that is not the purpose of this book; that is not the message I aim to deliver.

I think the first seeds for this idea were planted years ago when our daughter, Christy, was 10. One day she asked, "How come Grandmother Scarborough is 95 and she's not old?"

I remember saying, "Some people

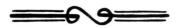

are old when they are 20, and some people are never old." Grandmother passed away peacefully at 96, but she was never old.

One of our favorite memories of Grandmother is how she would go to the nursing home to visit the "old folks"—most of whom were much younger in years than she was.

I've spent a lot of time visiting at assisted living facilities and nursing homes in recent years, and I've been taking notes on what my older friends have to say.

Ginny, one of the eldest of my interviewees made it to 100. She said, "I can't say I'm happy to have lived this long, but at least I got to see my great-granddaughter graduate from high school."

She put it a little more positively than Theda, who flatly stated, "I hate being this old," about three weeks

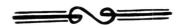

before her death at 95.

Ola Mae, who died at 96 said, "My nephew wants me to live to be 100, but I don't want to live that long." One week before her departure, Ola Mae said to me, "I'm ready to go when the Lord comes to get me, but I think I'm more ready than He is."

I'm reminded of a line from the movie *Grumpy Old Men* when two old guys heard that a friend of theirs had died from a heart attack in his sleep. "Lucky SOB," they agreed.

John, who was suffering with cancer and heart disease once told me, "I'm praying every day for a heart attack." He felt as if he had lived on borrowed time for 20 years, and he was tired.

I don't share these stories and sentiments lightly, but to show that there is a time when people tire of this earthly existence and decide it is time to go.

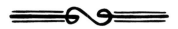

I remember the last time I went to visit Calva, a dear friend and mentor of mine. She had just turned 92, and more than once in the conversation she said, "My brother lived till 98 and my sister lived till 95, but I don't want to live that long."

She had suffered a stroke, and she was unable to continue the active lifestyle that she so enjoyed. She told her daughter, Cindy, "I wish I could have died in my prime—at 89."

Cindy and Calva both have a wonderful sense of humor, and we all three laughed when Cindy said, "Well, Mom, I guess you should have smoked."

If you feel as Faron Young and my brother do, that we should "live fast, love hard, die young, and leave a beautiful memory," perhaps you may think that this book is not for you. Actually, I think it is written just for you...

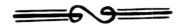

The special people mentioned here did live and love and leave us with precious memories and with valuable life lessons about how to live to enjoy all the days of our lives—no matter how many that may be.

"May you live a long life and DIE YOUNG." ~Cervantes

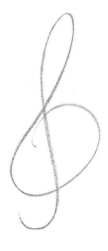

GuiDANCE:

What loving lessons and beautiful memories will you leave behind when your days on earth are done?

chapter 4

You Can't Keep a Good Woman Down!

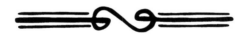

Maw, my maternal grandmother, aka Miss Ovie, is my "shero." As one of our family friends said, "Maw didn't just survive, she really thrived." Her attitude is one I choose to emulate. When she was 80, Maw fell and broke her hip and had to go to a nursing home for care.

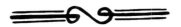

Christy heard this news about her great-grandmother and sighed, "When people go to nursing homes, they never get out."

Well, that was not the case with Miss Ovie! Maw said, "You can't keep a good woman down!" She followed doctor's orders, did her therapy, and after three months, went home and lived alone another 10 years, until she was 90. I can still see her dancin' with my daddy at her 90th birthday party.

Unlike her mother, Mommie, who fell and broke her hip and never walked again, Maw CHOSE to keep trying. She got up, "shook herself off," and intentionally kept going.

One day I was walking through Walgreens and I saw some little Beanie Baby Energizer Bunnies. When I spied those pink rabbits, I knew instantly that they were a symbol of my research. We've all seen the battery

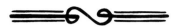

commercial with the tireless Energizer Bunny that keeps on going and going. Its perpetual motion reminds us to just keep putting one foot in front of the other and to not give up.

I remember a decision point in my mama, Dollie's, life. She had fallen and had bandages, seemingly, from head to toe. She was in her assisted living apartment sitting in a wheelchair—afraid to get up and walk again. After several serious falls, she was ready to confine herself to the safety of the wheelchair. Fear of falling had her paralyzed. I lovingly said, "Mama, we have two examples in our lives. We have Mommie, who fell and never walked again, and we have Maw, who fell and said, "You can't keep a good woman down!"

"Which one are you going to be like—Mommie or Maw? When you're gone, we're going to be talking about

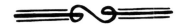

you, like we do them. What do you want us to say?"

She thought about it and said, "I want to be like Maw."

I am proud to tell you that Mama Dollie recovered from that fall and made a choice to keep going for several more years.

An interesting thing happened recently. I can only describe it as miraculous because it was so serendipitous.

I was invited to a local assisted living home to speak to the volunteers and residents on how we can live better longer. A number of them were folks I had already interviewed for my study, and they were interested to hear what I had learned so far.

I had my handy dandy Energizer Bunny on my dining room table next to my notes and planned to use it as a visual aid for my program. I didn't realize I had forgotten it at home until I was headed down the hall toward the meeting room. Just then, Marilyn, one of the residents who I knew well, came rolling by me in her wheelchair. She was carrying an Energizer Bunny exactly like mine! I said, "Marilyn, funny thing you should come rolling by with an Energizer Bunny. It reminds me that I didn't bring the one I planned to use. Could I use yours?"

She flashed a huge smile and said, "Of course, I was just bringing this to show my friends. My granddaughter, Kristen, sent it to me and said, "Grandmother, you're the Energizer Bunny. You just keep going and going!"

Marilyn, Maw, and Mama Dollie are all great examples that you can't keep a good woman down when she makes an intentional decision to keep on going—to keep on keeping on—to keep on dancin'.

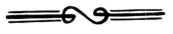

Don't Quit

Author Unknown

When things go wrong, as they
*   sometimes will,*
When the road you're trudging
*   seems all uphill,*
When the funds are low and the
*   debts are high*
And you want to smile, but you
*   have to sigh,*
When care is pressing you down
*   a bit,*
Rest if you must, but don't you
*   quit.*
Life is queer with its twists and
*   turns,*
As every one of us sometimes
*   learns,*
And many a failure turns about,
When he might have won had
*   he stuck it out.*
Don't give up though the pace
*   seems slow,*
You may succeed with another
*   blow.*
Success is failure turned inside
*   out,*

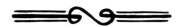

The silver tint of the clouds of doubt,
And you never can tell how close you are,
It may be near when it seems so far;
So stick to the fight when you're hardest hit
It's when things seem worse that you must not quit.

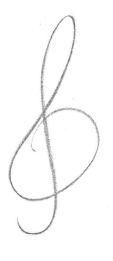

GuiDANCE:

Can you think of a time when you or someone you love had to make a conscious choice to keep on going?

43

chapter 5

I Wanted to Go; I Went, and I Had a Good Time

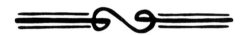

When Maw was 93, she was living at the Monument Hill Nursing home and still taking part in the activities offered. A field trip to the Blue Bell Ice Cream factory was planned, and she signed up to go. Aunt Doris, her primary care-giver, protectively said, "Now, Maw, you don't need to

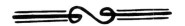

go on that field trip." She was thinking, *You might fall, and you won't remember it anyway*.

On the day of the excursion, Aunt Doris wasn't around, so Maw got on the bus and went on the tour. She loved escaping for a while and especially enjoyed free samples of Homemade Vanilla Blue Bell afterwards. The next day, when her daughter, Doris, heard about the decision, she said, "Why, Maw, I thought you weren't gonna go on that field trip!"

Maw's words have become my mantra. "I wanted to go; I went, and I had a good time."

It was my honor to speak at Maw's funeral when she passed away at 96, and I shared that story with those who gathered to celebrate the life of Miss Ovie—Ovie Parker Lueders Blankenburg—Maw.

She left us with many life lessons

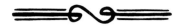

and that was one of them: "I wanted to go; I went, and I had a good time."

Several years ago I hosted a New Mexico Red Hat Lady Retreat at a beautiful mountain resort, and that was the theme of the weekend. In memory of Maw, we gathered to have a good time...and we did!

Her story reminds us not to make decisions out of fear and not to let someone else make decisions for us out of fear. She followed her own inner prompting to go—to accept the invitation for a day of fun. Fear of falling or forgetting did not deter Maw. She wanted to go; she went, and she had a good time and left me with that legacy.

Although Maw may have forgotten that day as time went by and her memory faded, I have not forgotten. I've learned from her example, and it is my mission to share this life lesson

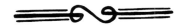

from Miss Ovie with my daughter, Christy, my granddaughter, Aubrey, and anyone else who wants to have a good time in life.

> **"For God has not given us the spirit of fear, but of power, and of love, and of a sound mind."**
> **2 Timothy 1:7**

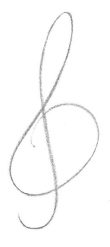

GuiDANCE:

What life lessons can you learn from your grandmother or grandfather?

chapter 6

Get Up Every Day and Put on Your Face

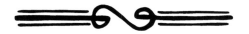

Another life lesson from Maw passed along to my mama and me was: "Get up every day, get dressed, and put on your face, because you never know who's gonna come to the door."

She taught us not to slouch around the house looking tacky and tired. Some may not see the significance of

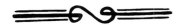

this advice, but it is profound. When we look our best, we just feel better. If we wake up, comb our hair, and put on makeup and some "foo foo" powder, our attitude is enhanced. If we have on clean clothes and comfortable shoes, we are ready for any expected or unexpected adventure. We are prepared, feel prettier, and are more productive as we perform our daily tasks. When guys get up and shower and shave and put in their teeth, they are less likely to be couch potatoes.

I'm reminded of my beautiful friend, Emma Lee. In her later years she lived in an assisted living complex that was on my way to town. Often I would stop by, knock on her door and ask, "Would you like to go...?" and before I could finish the sentence, she said, "Yes," and grabbed her purse.

She was dressed and ready for action. We had many memorable times—just being together. I am so

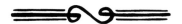

glad she accepted my invitations.

Dorothy was also always impeccably dressed. In the years I knew her, she was in assisted living and later in a nursing home, but she always looked noticeably better than others up and down the hall. She told me that her mother taught her to take pride in her appearance, and she heeded that advice all the days of her life. I smile as I remember what she said as the ambulance wheeled her off to the hospital for the last time. A friend of hers stopped by just as the EMTs were rolling her out the door. Tootie asked, "Oh, Dorothy, are you all right?"

Dorothy said, "No, I am so sick... Does my hair look ok?"

When Maw quit putting on her makeup, we knew that the end was near. Mama spent her last three days of life asleep, but that's about the

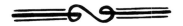

only time I can remember when she didn't get up and get dressed and put her best *face* forward. I'm grateful to these women—Maw, Mama, Emma Lee, and Dorothy, who were good examples to me through the seemingly simple act of getting up every day and being intentional about "putting on their faces."

Before publication, I shared this manuscript with my friend Carol and after reading this chapter, she wrote back and told me about her mother-in-law, Rose. She shared that Rose always said that she did not want to die in her sleep because she wouldn't have her makeup on. I can relate...

Carol's response of remembering her loved one and sharing her story is something that I hope will happen as others read this book. If you have thoughts, observations, or stories that you want to relate to me, please send them to kateasbill@gmail.com or visit

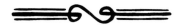

our website at: <u>www.startdancin.com</u>

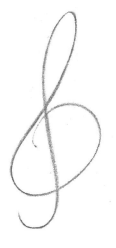

GuiDANCE:

Are you putting your best face forward?

chapter 7

Go and Do While You Can

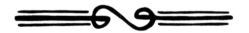

Iwas sitting in the lab at the hospital when I overheard this thought-provoking conversation. An older gentleman said, "Go and do while you can! We had lots of plans for after we retired, but now we just have to decide—'Do we want to go to the doctor, hospital, or pharmacy first?"

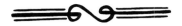

He was giving this timely advice to his younger friend who was about to retire.

As I've visited with older friends through the years, there seems to be a recurring theme in their advice. "Honey, go and do while you can," they tell me. Some say it with regret or remorse that they didn't go and do things while they were physically able. Others speak from experience and advise me to travel and see the world while I can. The message is the same from both groups: **"Go and do; make a lot of happy memories; take a lot of pictures!"**

Martha often mentions the happy times that she and Henry had camping in Colorado. They went every summer for many years. Aunt Doris and Uncle Gene flew many times to Mexico and to England and, once, to France to see the Eiffel Tower. She recalled a favorite memory of taking her mother,

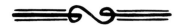

my grandmother, Maw, to Hawaii. Mildred has many memories of when she and James and my parents traveled together to Branson, Hawaii, and other delightful destinations. There are photo albums filled with special memories of good times shared with fun friends and family.

Margaret and Norman are in their late eighties, and they still go camping for several months each summer. They enjoy the company of old friends at a beautiful campground that they have frequented for over thirty years. Newell, who is nearly ninety, has someone else drive and park his motor home, but with these adaptations, he can still do what he loves.

Stories of shared experiences are told and retold when old friends get together or talk on the phone. Reminiscing about past experiences that were positive and recollecting happy days when all was well, can bring joy

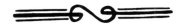

later on in life. Pictures and journals help to keep the memories alive. Take pictures. You'll be glad you did.

To "go and do" does not necessarily mean leaving town. It can also refer to going and doing things "in your own back yard." I've been watching two wonderful widow ladies in our community. Both of them are in their eighties and still going strong. It seems that everywhere I go, I see one or both of them—at restaurants, at church, or at community events. Earlier this month my daughter, Christy, and I went to a Clint Black concert, and there they were—having a big time. They invited us to sit with them. Evolyn explained why they had chosen the wide aisle seats and how they had parked near the side entrance for easy access. They were intentional about accommodations that could be made for safety and enjoyment. I saw them later that week at the

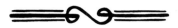

high school football game—cheering on the team. They talked about how they enjoy going to the senior center meal site each weekday for food and fellowship. We spoke with concern about a mutual friend who has been suffering with depression, and they talked about how that friend could be invited, included, and encouraged to join them there.

Each Sunday I see Evolyn at church and Mary Elizabeth at Community Bible Study on Wednesday. They always have a big smile and a friendly hug for me. Both of these ladies have had health challenges in recent times, but Evolyn didn't let a serious fall keep her down, and Mary Elizabeth hasn't let skin cancer keep her from keepin' on! I want to be like them when I grow up.

The other day I heard someone say: "All Grandma does is sit on the couch and Grandpa waits on her." Another

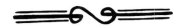

person expressed concern over her significant other who only wants to sit in his recliner and watch TV. Health issues, disabilities, and accidents can cause us to have to sit on the couch for a while, but we don't have to stay there! Make a determined effort to get up and go and do while you can.

"Don't let what you can't do keep you from doing what you can." ~Sign at Senior Center

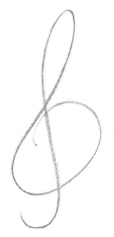

GuiDANCE:

Are there places you want to go and things you want to do?

chapter 8

Don't Worry, Be Happy

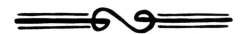

There is a catchy tune called "Don't Worry, Be Happy" that has a simple, but meaningful, message for all of us.

We have a choice each day as to whether we will worry or not, and whether we will be happy or not. We choose our own "whether—weather."

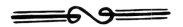

We can wake every morning and decide to be happy. Each day before getting out of bed we can greet the day with a smile and say with Psalm 118:24, "This is the day that the Lord has made. Let us rejoice and be glad in it!" There is power in this Scripture and in this attitude. This Scripture and others can give us guidance for daily living. It has been said that there are 365 Scriptures in the Bible that say, "Fear not," and instruct us not to worry.

My precious mother, Dollie, was a worrier. She had many wonderful characteristics that I admire, and I want to be like her in many ways, but not in that one. Once she was worrying about something and I said, "Mama, sometimes you worry so much about tomorrow that you can't enjoy today."

My daddy had his first open heart surgery at age 60 and then lived on borrowed time for twenty more years.

He led a full and active life, and they had a great time together. She loved him dearly and couldn't imagine having a happy life without him. Although she rarely spoke of it, I know that she lived in dread of the day when he would be dead. She was one of the most caring and loving people who ever lived, and perhaps, because of that deep love for Daddy and her family and friends, she worried.

I've heard that "our strengths carried to an extreme can become our weaknesses," and I feel that is true.

You may have heard someone say, "I was worried to death." I believe it happens; some people have literally worried themselves to death.

My maternal grandmother, Kate, who I was named after, died 7 months before I was born. She was only 63, and her hair was white as snow. I've been told that she was a wonderful

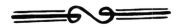

Christian woman, with wit and charm, and a keen sense of humor. I wish I could have known her. She passed away 13 months after my daddy, her oldest son, returned home from World War II. Someone in the family told me that she was so worried about the safety of her precious son that it made her sick. I don't doubt it. I have all the letters Daddy wrote home to her during the war, and there is a recurring theme throughout—"Don't worry about me. I'll be all right." He was. She wasn't. It is my belief that she worried herself to death.

I know that saying, "Don't worry, be happy," is easier said than done, but I do believe that if we are prone to worry, we can make a conscious choice to monitor our thoughts and to intentionally change that habit. Worrying is in my genes, and that tendency can creep up on me if I am not vigilant. I try to monitor my

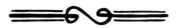

thoughts, and if negativity sneaks in, I literally "change the channel." I learned this from a clever friend many years ago.

I put my hand up next to my head and pretend to turn a knob: changing the channel from one of *fear* to one of *faith*.

Works for me. Give it a try.

"And which of you by worrying can add a single hour to his life span?" Luke 12:25

"Be so happy that when others look at you they become happy too." ~Thereasa Ramsey

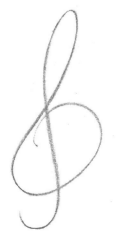

GuiDANCE:

Do you need to "change the channel" from fear to faith?

chapter 9

How Come We're Born if We're Just Gonna Die Again?

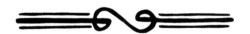

One of the saddest things I have ever heard someone say is, "I don't have a thing in the world to do." She was sincere when she said it, and at that time I believed her. Beth was feeling down and depressed and couldn't see past herself. Outside the door of her private room at the nurs-

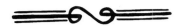

ing facility, there were others down the hall who could have used a smile, a hug, or a friendly hello. She could have held someone's hand and whispered a prayer of hope or help. Her mind was still sharp, and we could have considered some options together. She was an accomplished pianist, and maybe we could have found a piano for her to play. That would have served three purposes—lifting her own spirits, adding some sweet sounds to the silent corridors of the facility, and brightening the mood of both residents and caregivers. "Coulda, woulda, shoulda," more sad words...

Although it is too late to correct that situation, reflecting upon that story can give us "food for thought" for future action. It brings to mind the power of *purpose*. I've come to believe that we arrive on earth with a purpose in life, and if we're still here, our mission is not complete. This poem,

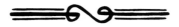

which I first heard at a banquet to honor volunteers at a nursing home, is a reminder that we do not outlive our purpose:

"Someone Needs You"

If you're feeling sad and lonely,
There seems nothing you can
do,
Just take courage and remember
There is someone needing you.

You were created for a purpose,
For a part of God's great plan
Bear ye one another's burdens,
So fulfill Christ's law to man.

Are you father, son, or
daughter?
You've a work none else can do.
Are you husband, wife, or
mother?
There is someone needing you.

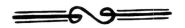

If perhaps in bed you're lying
You can smile or press the hand
Of the one who tells his story;
He will know you understand.

There are many sad and lonely,
And discouraged, not a few,
Who a little cheer are needing,
And there's someone needing
you.

Someone needs your faith and
courage;
Someone needs your love and
prayer;
Someone needs your inspiration,
Thus to help their cross to bear.

Do not think your work is ended,
There is much that you can do.
And as long as you're on earth,
There is someone needing YOU."

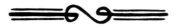

Thinking about life's purpose brings to mind something significant that happened many years ago. Jimmy was just seven, a second grader in my class, when he asked me, "How come we're born, if we're just going to die again?" I was a young teacher at that point in time, but I recognized the importance of both his question and my answer. Little Jimmy had recently suffered the tragic loss of his younger sister, and I'm sure that's what prompted him to ask me that age-old question.

I don't remember exactly what I said, but it seemed to satisfy him on that day. He has probably continued to contemplate that question through the thirty-something years that have passed since our paths first crossed. I have.

As I recall my answer to my precious student, it seems to me that I told Jimmy that life is like a school,

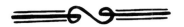

and that there are tests and trials we have to face as we learn life lessons. I told him that we come to earth with a purpose, a job to do while we are here. (Ephesians 2:10 "For we are God's workmanship, created in Christ Jesus to do good works, which God prepared in advance for us to do.")

I really didn't address his under-lying question about why his little sister died so young. I didn't know then, and I don't know now. Jimmy and I, and many others, will have to ask our Heavenly Father about that someday. He's much smarter than Jimmy's second grade teacher.

I still believe we all come to this planet with a purpose—something we can do that no one else can ac-complish. There are trials and tests along the way, and how we respond will determine our forward progress toward our goal. I have come to know that we are not in this life alone. God

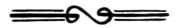

sends us helpers and teachers—both seen and unseen, to tutor us in the school of life. We also have the power of prayer, and we can call upon the Holy Spirit when we need help along the way.

I'm reminded of Calva, who was confined to her home and her chair, but continued to say, "I pay and I pray." She was faithful in her finances, and she used her money to help her family and several philanthropic causes. She prayed always for the needs of others. When her health declined and she had to slow down and finally sit down, she still found a purpose—something meaningful to do.

No matter what our age, our lives can be enriched if we find ways to serve others. My mama, Dollie, was a master of caring for and about those she knew. When asked for a quote or Scripture to put on her square for

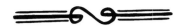

a memorial quilt, I chose, "Always Thinking of Others." That was how she lived her life. It was her passion, her purpose, her legacy—her cause beyond herself.

Edna, age 90, told me, "I thank the Lord every day for letting me live a purposeful life." She said, "I never thought I'd be a widow. Morris was always in such good condition, but he had an accident and never recovered from that." She told me that after he died, she asked the Lord, "Why did you leave me here?" And that she heard the answer, "as clear as I'm talking to you, He said, 'I'm not through with you yet. Go and have a good time.'" She continued, "I took the Lord at His word."

She has traveled to many places that she had never seen, taking along different family members. She continued to play the piano and organ for Sunday services and looked for other

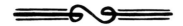

ways to serve the Lord. For fourteen years she got to play the magnificent pipe organ at New Mexico Military Institute. She just "gave the keys back" last year.

Edna loves to read and after I told her about my interest in pro-active aging, she said, "I got something in the mail yesterday that you would like." She related that the article about longevity from the Duke Medical Center said, "People who have a purpose are more likely to live longer, healthier lives."[2] Edna summed it up this way:

"You always have to have a carrot out there to keep you going."

What's your carrot? What is your passion—your purpose? We were sent to earth with something special to do. The happiest people are those who figure out what it is.

As the research article that Edna

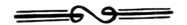

shared stated, "One benefit of find-ing your purpose early in life is that you can live healthier longer."[2] If you are yet to discover your purpose, try doing what Edna did. Pray to know why you're here, and then *listen*.

> **"Seek God's will in all you do, and He will show you the path to take." Proverbs 3:6**

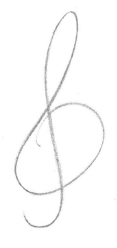

GuiDANCE:

Have you tried prayer?

What is your "carrot," your purpose, your mission, your reason for being?

chapter 10

Visiting the Olderly

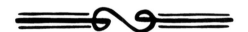

One day at church, Betty stood to share an anecdote about a little boy who proudly told her about his Sunday School class project. "We're going to visit the 'olderly,'" he said with a toothy grin.

Is there an "olderly" person who would be blessed by a visit from you?

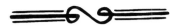

Think of someone today who would relish time in your presence, and, I promise, you are the one who will be blessed.

Vernon's parents, Tom and Olivia, were faithful to visit their friends who were confined to the nursing home. They followed the example of her mother, Grandmother S., who made regular visits to the "old folks home" (as she called it) until she was 95. My mother, Dollie, and her friends used to visit the shut-ins in their community, and she served as a sponsor for the Seasoned Citizen Camp, long before she was a senior herself. I am proud of this legacy of love left by these thoughtful family members.

The other day I was at a nursing home when I saw an old friend of mine who was there to teach a Bible study. He stopped by for a quick hello in Ed's room where I was visiting. While he was there, he shared how his ministry

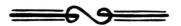

to the "olderly" began. Jim said that when his father, Herb, was in failing health and needed constant care, he was admitted to a nursing home. Jim found himself getting upset because no one else was coming to visit Herb. He related to me that after he prayed about the situation, "The Lord said, 'How often did you come before your dad was here?'" Jim took heed.

He greeted my friend, Ed, and said, "I'll be back. I try to come out here most every day."

Jim and I have a heritage of concern and love for the elderly. Twelve years ago when I first met Jim's dad, Herb, he was a daily visitor at the home where his wife, Lois, was a resident. On his way to see the love of his life, he would stop to see and converse with others along the way— sharing the latest news and a laugh or two. Residents in both assisted living and the nursing home looked forward

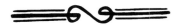

to the pleasure of his company. Jim learned that lesson from his dad and is now following in Herb's footsteps.

Jim's ministry to the elderly and disabled will have eternal consequences. Last week, he and I were talking to our precious friend, Faith, when Jim asked her to tell me her big news. Faith's face was beaming as she looked up at me from her wheelchair and smiled, saying, "I got baptized!" God has blessed Faith and others through His servant, Jim.

As I was leaving that day, after a visit with my dear friend Frances I assured her that I would be back soon. "Good," she smiled, "I thrive on that."

If you are searching for a "cause beyond yourself," I recommend volunteering at a local nursing home or regularly visiting the "olderly" men and women from your church or

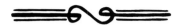

community. You'll be glad you did.

"I have learned that the best classroom in the world is at the feet of an elderly person."
~Andy Rooney

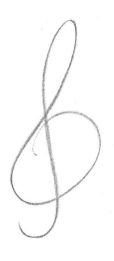

GuiDANCE:

Is there someone waiting on a visit or a call from you?

Could you bless someone and brighten their day and help her or him to thrive?

·

chapter *11*

If I Sat Down at the Piano, the World Went Away

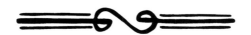

When I met Ida, she lived in the Memory Care Center, but there were some things she didn't have any trouble remembering. My primary reason for going to see her was to share communion with her as part of our church's ministry to shut-ins. She seemed to understand the

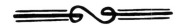

significance of the sacrament, and she was appreciative of my attention.

After we shared some sacred moments, I decided to stay a while and get to know her better. We visited for a few minutes, talking about life and love. At one point, I asked, "Is there anything you would have done differently?"

Without hesitating she replied, "I wouldn't have married the same guy."

"Really? How long were you married?"

"Twenty-eight years."

"Did you get a divorce?"

"No, but I had my *music*. If I sat down at the piano, the world went away."

Her memory seemed to be working fine as she recalled a tough time of life. It seemed to me that in addition to communion, we had shared

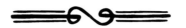

something else of significance. Her revelation of how her love for music had carried her through many years in a bad marriage spoke volumes to me.

I was reminded of another earlier conversation with my dear friend Dorothy. She shared, "I don't know what I would have done after my husband died if it hadn't been for my music."

There seemed to be a connection between how music helped Ida sustain her spirit while in a rocky relationship and how music helped Dorothy carry on with life after the loss of her loved one.

Ida was the music teacher of a man I know, and he continues to love music and sings in the church choir every Sunday. I'm certain there are countless others who were positively influenced by her passion for piano

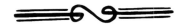

and singing. No doubt, music now sustains some of them through tough times.

Dorothy had a beautiful voice and after her husband's death, she joined a group called "Women of Note." For fifteen years they traveled up and down the California coast singing beautiful harmony. That experience was one she relished and loved to recall all the days of her life.

Although she was older when I met her, she showed me the pictures and told me tales of their travels. In her room in assisted living, which just happened to be the same room Mama had once occupied, Dorothy had quite a collection of beautiful musical tapes—recordings of herself singing with others.

Her favorites, by far, were those she had of herself and her beloved brother, Theron, happily harmonizing.

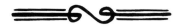

They had a close and loving relationship and their shared love for music
probably strengthened that bond.
In her latter years, after Theron was
gone, she would listen to those tapes,
sing along, and, I'm sure, the world
went away.

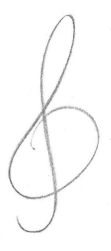

GuiDANCE:

What activities do you
enjoy enough to make the
world go away?

chapter *12*

We Don't Stop Playing Because We Grow Old; We Grow Old Because We Stop Playing

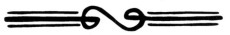

We celebrated Mimi and Tom's 64th anniversary along with Christmas, never knowing they would both be gone before spring arrived. She was 87, and he was 96, and they still lived in their cozy Texas home. Everyday they would play several games of dominoes, and I believe that

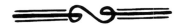

is one of the things that allowed them to stay put and stay married.

Mimi kept all the tally sheets in a handy-dandy notebook. We saved the neatly written record as a reminder of the 1,164 games they played during their last year of life together.

We smile as we remember Tom-Tom's standard answer when asked who usually won. "It's kind of hard to beat the scorekeeper," he often quipped. Who won or lost was not what was important. What *was* important was that they kept playing—together. It was a way of staying connected, keeping their minds sharp, and passing the time.

I'm reminded of a country music song by Trace Atkins that says, "She thinks we're just fishin'." A dad is reflecting on the beauty and benefits of doing things together—like fishing with his daughter. Dominoes is what

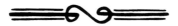

Mimi and Tom-Tom did, but there are many other ways to play together.

Following the example of Vernon's parents, Mimi and Tom-Tom, Vernon and I learned to play mah-jongg and two kinds of rummy. We also play Scrabble. Many evenings are spent playing together or with friends. I keep the scores for each year in a little notebook, and he agrees with his dad, "It's kinda hard to beat the scorekeeper." But, he is ahead...

As I have interviewed people for this project, I have observed that those seniors who are continuing to regularly play games such as bridge, rummy, mah-jongg, Mexican train, bunco, hand and foot, dominoes, and golf with friends are usually mentally alert and socially connected. Verna and Mary love to play bridge, and Joe and Reid meet weekly with their poker buddies—as they have for about 50 years. J.T. and Vernon

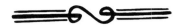

have fun playing golf together several times a week. Although the mental and physical exercise is important, the coming together for fellowship is equally so. It may appear that they're just playin', but much more is going on.

My mother and daddy and their friends loved to play a domino game called "42." I have few regrets in life, but there are a couple of things that I would do differently. When Mama said, "Let's play 42," I wish I would have done it. The good news is that in the last few months, I have taken "42" lessons and I will never pass up another invitation to play!

My daddy loved to fish. I didn't go along, and he quit inviting me. You see, I thought it was "just fishin'," and I missed opportunities for precious time together. I've heard that most of our regrets are not for things we did, but for things we didn't do.

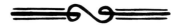

Invitations unaccepted can haunt us if we allow it.

Be intentional about learning to play some games and invite your spouse, your family, or some fun friends to "come out and play."

As George Bernard Shaw believed, "We don't stop playing because we grow old; we grow old because we stop playing."

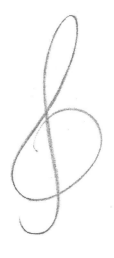

GuiDANCE:

Who could you invite over to play?

chapter 13

Different Strokes for Different Folks

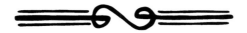

Vernon and I were on our way to a church picnic when I said, "I'm going to find the oldest people there and visit with them." After placing my fried chicken with the other pot-luck offerings and greeting those who had gathered, I made a bee-line for Erma, the matriarch of the group. She was

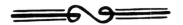

a spunky little woman who talked fast and moved quickly despite her advanced age. She proudly announced that she was 94 although I didn't ask.

After we had visited for a few minutes, I told her about my interest in pro-active aging. I said, "It seems to me that you've done something right to be thriving at 94. What's your secret?"

After thinking for a second or two, she stated, "I didn't smoke, I didn't drink, and I didn't go with fellows that did. When I went out with a fellow, I watched-that-glass. If he drank too much, I made him take me home, and I never went out with him again!"

She shared other facts, but her philosophy about not smoking and moderate drinking stuck with me. Sometime later I repeated what she told me to Flo, an outgoing octogenarian, and Flo said, "How boring!"

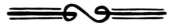

She added, "I like to drink milk, but sometimes I put a little whiskey in it." She smiled and continued to tell me how she and her little dog, Bitsy, have "happy hour" every day at 5:00. "Bitsy always lets me know when it's time, and we drink out of the same glass." I thought, *Different strokes for different folks...*

I remembered Thomas who told me, with a twinkle in his eye, that his secret to longevity was "whiskey and wild women." I think he was pulling my leg; he was known for his fun sense of humor—which was probably the real reason he made it to 95½.

Erma's decisions not to smoke, not to drink excessively, and not to marry a man who drank too much may have saved her from years of heartache. Her comments caused me to ponder personal decisions I've made through the years about abstinence and moderation. I thought of others who made different choices about drugs and alcohol and how their lives may have been happier and healthier and longer had they not made certain choices along the way.

Two of my uncles were killed in World War II in their twenties, and that was a horrible tragedy for our family. Two other beloved uncles died in their seventies from lung cancer, probably caused by decades of smoking, and that was equally tragic.

If you are still smoking, please stop. Now. If you have tried stopping unsuccessfully, try again. Nicotine patches have helped some people. One of my friends was able to break the habit by using Chantix, and several others were able to taper off, and finally quit with the help of electronic cigarettes. I know that the verdict is still out on the safety of e-cigs, but they have helped some to stop smoking. An addiction to cigarettes is a

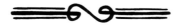

hard habit to break, but you can do it!

If you have never smoked, don't start.

Alcohol in excess has destroyed countless marriages, careers, and lives. I am saddened to think of those I've known who abused alcohol and drugs and didn't live long enough to see the successes of their children or get to hold the hands of their grand-children. Moderation or abstinence might have made a difference.

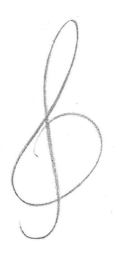

GuiDANCE:

Are there any unhealthy habits you need to change?

chapter 14

We All Know Better Than We Do

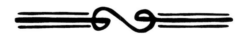

When I went to see Ruth, I got more than I bargained for. I went to see my old friend to ask for her advice on how to live better longer. Ruth lives alone, still drives, is active in church and other organizations, and stays in touch daily with several of her close friends. Her mind

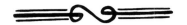

is sharp, and she says what she thinks. I always enjoy her company.

After we spent about an hour talking about her life and what she had learned in her 90+ years on earth, she offered me some tea. As we walked into the kitchen to get our drinks, she stopped suddenly, turned around, pointed her finger at me, and bluntly asked, "Kate, what are you going to do about that weight?"

I was somewhat taken aback but should not have been surprised. I have noticed that when some people reach 90, they realize they can get away with saying anything that pops into their heads.

Of course, in my reading and research on positive aging, I have heard the importance of maintaining a healthy weight and the harmful effects of added pounds. I have known Ruth since I was a young, "skinny little thing," and that is no longer the case. Her forthright manner is one of the things I have always admired about Ruth, but still, I was not expecting her pointed question. It was a good question, and one that deserved an answer and some action. I'm not sure what I said—probably something like, "We all know better than we do."

She continued, "What did you have for lunch?"

"Salad," I answered.

"Without dressing?" she queried.

I shook my head, "Nope—Ranch dressing."

"No dressing," she advised, "or bread. You've got to watch the sugar too," she added. "I eat carrots and celery sticks for supper."

I laughed and said, "I know; you're right." I meant it when I said, "Thanks for reminding me. I'll do better."

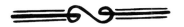

I smiled as I got into my car to leave. The personal question, "Kate, what are you going to do about that weight?" was perfectly in line with the purpose of my visit. After I left her home, I was prompted to contemplate losing weight. At that time I had been interviewing people for about nine years and asking them advice about what can be done to live better longer. Although no one but Ruth had given me such accurate personal advice, I had already made many life style changes and choices. I knew I needed to heed her advice.

The next day I had lunch with my friend Vicki at our favorite Mexican food place. After thinking for twenty-four hours about Ruth's advice to lose some weight, and having carrot sticks and celery for supper the night before, I sat staring at the menu.

I decided—stuffed avocado salad. No dressing.

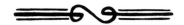

As the waitress approached, Vicki said, "I always get Guadalajara."

"Me too, I confessed."

We ordered two.

I was thinking, "We all know better than we do..."

We did skip the sopapillas.

I vowed to myself, *Next time, I'll have salad.*

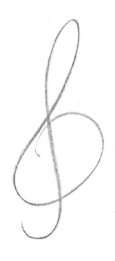

GuiDANCE:

What are you going to do about that weight?

chapter 15

It's Just What the Dr. Ordered

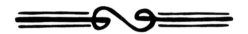

Iengaged several doctors in conversation concerning the advice they give their patients and what they believe can be done to live better longer.

Dr. B said, "Pick your parents and grandparents carefully," indicating his belief in the importance of genes. There has always been a debate about which factor plays the larger role in longevity—genetics or life choices. While genes are important, I fall into the camp of those who believe personal choices make a bigger difference in the quality of life than genes.

Dr. W, who was confined to a wheel chair due to complications from diabetes, looked at me sadly—shaking his head as he said, "Don't get diabetes." While some of us are pre-disposed to that disease because of heredity, life style choices have been shown to help with prevention of this dreaded disease. Daily decisions also make a huge difference in quality of life if someone is diagnosed with diabetes. This alarming statement in an article in the Blues Healthline magazine caught my attention: "More than 120,000 New Mexicans have diabetes, but only 84,000 know they have it." [3]

Another scary statistic reported in the Oct. 2014 AARP Bulletin is this:

"The ratio of Americans 65 and older with diabetes is 1 in 4." Dr. Daniel Lorber, director of the Division of Endocrinology at New York Hospital Queens said, "Being overweight and sedentary increase the odds of both type 2 diabetes and heart disease." But Dr. Robert Lustig, who also specializes in diabetes research, cautions, "It's a dangerous myth that type 2 diabetes is exclusively caused by being overweight or obese." He concluded, "The bottom line is: being overweight or obese is a good reason to be tested for type 2 diabetes, but being thin is no excuse for ignoring your risk."

Dr. Lorber, who sees many patients with diabetes states, "As physicians we counsel, we coach, we prescribe, we cheerlead. But the only person who treats diabetes is the person who has it." [4]

Healthy life-style choices like con-

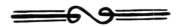

suming less, moving more, and taking medication if necessary are all changes that can make a big difference in the prevention or management of diabetes. More helpful information on this topic is readily available from your physician and on the diabetes. org website.

I asked Dr. K what factors he felt could improve quality of life. He quickly said, "The three W's—water, weight, and walking." He had clearly been espousing these ideas for years. He added, "I tell people to drink lots of good, clean water, but not just any water. I have to remove a lot of kidney and gall stones, and I believe they are primarily caused from the minerals in our drinking water. You need to install a reverse osmosis water filtration system in your home." I took his advice and that is what I got Vernon for Christmas that year.

Dr. K also stated strongly the need

for walking regularly for exercise, and the importance of maintaining a healthy weight. His advice about walking regularly is supported by research and is often touted as a key to a healthy life. His emphasis on watching your weight for maximum health benefits is mentioned in almost every article on health care and longevity. His recommendations prompted me to join Curves, and later, to join Weight Watchers.

I've seen numerous doctors on TV talking about the power of positive attitudes. Dr. B reported that research has shown that those with a better attitude live longer. It has also been shown that the optimists are happier and enjoy each day of life more than the pessimists. We have a daily choice—opt for optimism!

Dr. R was on the news talking about how to live to be one hundred. He smiled and quipped, "First, live

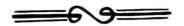

to be 99, and then, don't fall for a year." Falls are often the "downfall" of senior citizens and can lead to their demise. Dr. R offered these suggestions for fall prevention: "Wear sturdy shoes, use a cane if needed, and do not multi-task while walking." It has been my observation that the old saying, "Pride goes before a fall" can be true if people refuse to carry a needed cane because of vanity.

Dr. Harold Koenig, who is one of the world's top experts on faith and longevity recently conducted a major study on faith, healing, and prayer, and he concluded that people who are religious, people of faith, can add 7 to 14 years to their lives. The topic of religion and health is one of interest to me and to many. If you want to learn more about Dr. Koenig's research, Google his name and read about this timely topic. The majority of the people I have interviewed, observed, and want to emulate are people of deep faith, and they believe that religion, spirituality, church attendance, and prayer have made a profound difference in their lives. Dr. Koenig's research seems to support my personal observations that faith, prayer, and connection to a church community are correlated with fuller, happier, longer lives.[5]

In the past ten years, I have read hundreds of articles and books on health and aging. Other people read novels, I read this stuff. I find it fascinating. I hope you do too. Much of it is repeated and reworded and reiterated, and the reason for that is—it's the truth!

This conversation sums up what I have come to believe: When I told Dr. J about my research on pro-active aging, he said, "The research is in. It's all there. We just have to do it!" You know what to do.

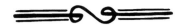

Start today. Stick with it for the rest of your life. It's just what the doctor ordered!

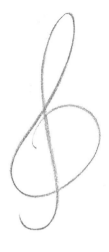

GuiDANCE:

Are there things you know you could be doing to help you live better longer?

chapter *16*

Exercise – Just Do It

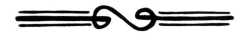

Years ago, I was driving to work and listening to Paul Harvey on the radio when I heard him say, "Walking decreases the chances of death by fifty percent." That comment caught my attention, and as I mulled it over in my mind, I realized something was missing. Later on that day, I heard the report again and caught the rest of the story, with this clarification: "Research has shown that *walking for exercise, three times a week for thirty minutes,* reduces the chances of *early death* by fifty percent." That made more sense.

I wish I had taken it to heart and started walking regularly back then. Whatever age you are now, just do it! Walking is the easiest and cheapest form of exercise. Many books and articles have been written about the benefits, but all it really takes is a decision and a pair of sturdy shoes. A treadmill and shots in your knees might be helpful, but do whatever it takes to begin exercising regularly.

You may prefer another form of exercise, but the bottom line is: Keep active. Keep fit. Keep moving. Find something that works for you—something you enjoy—something that fits with your age and stage of life. Set

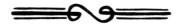

an app on your phone for a daily reminder. Start now. Stick with it.

A physical therapist told me that her professor said that if he could invent an "exercise pill," it would be the most widely used medication of all times and that it would do more good than any other pill ever prescribed. He stated that "an exercise pill would produce the most benefits for the most diagnoses of any prescription on the market today."

The bad news is—there is no such pill. The good news is—by making a decision to be intentional about exercise, we can "add years to our life and life to our years."[6]

Dr. V, an orthopedic surgeon, told Vernon and me that he believes riding a stationary bike is the best form of exercise. Dr. V said that as he was putting shots into Vernon's knees so he can continue to golf with friends, to hunt with our grandson, and to train for an annual hike in the Grand Canyon with my brothers, Perry and Ronnie. I have observed that having a goal of hiking 17.5 miles in the Grand Canyon keeps them all going year after year. None of them wants to be the one who says, "I can't go again this year." A little friendly competition between brothers ages 65-71 encourages them to stay in shape year round.

Last year Vernon sported a shirt that said, "Down is optional; up is mandatory." They made it out in the early afternoon, triumphant, happy, and in better condition than some half their age. Vernon and Ronnie have made the trek six times, and Perry has hiked it fourteen. These ambitious senior citizens are exercising every day in preparation for next year and looking forward to making more special memories. The

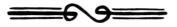

Grand Canyon adventure has become a challenging tradition enjoyed by three generations of our family. I am proud of my husband and brothers who are an inspiration to their kids and grandkids—including our son, Corey, daughter-in-law, Cassandra, and grandson, Addison.

Clara, who lived to be 93, would have agreed with Dr. V. about the value of riding a stationary bicycle. She was faithful about riding her bike each day for years, which was verified on the bicycle odometer that registered over 10,000 miles. Clara's consistent exercise of choice made a noticeable difference later on in her life. At one point, her hip broke, but she quickly recovered and continued to walk, well until her 93rd year of life. I smile as I remember how she would walk quickly down the hall, holding her walker above the floor. The doctor told her to get a walker

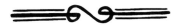

for support and balance, so she obediently carried it around with her.

I've found that riding my stationary bike as I watch the daily news is something that works for me. It has become a beneficial habit that I enjoy. As of today, I have recorded 2322.7 miles since I became intentional about riding regularly. That is like riding from my home in New Mexico almost all the way to Augusta, Maine! My goal is to catch up with Clara.

Some insist that "swimming is the kindest sport"—an ideal, low-impact aerobic exercise that uses all the major muscle groups.[7] Elizabeth would agree. She is 108 and lived alone until she was 107. When asked the secret to her long, healthy life, she related how she swam regularly for over forty years. She and several friends met each weekday morning at the natatorium and began their day with a dip in the pool. Elizabeth continued this practice until well into her 90s. The buddy system was also beneficial for this group of ladies. Elizabeth's daughter told me that if one of them was not planning to go, the others would encourage her to stick with the program. It took dedication to continue swimming regularly for four decades. They probably didn't intend to set any records, but day after day, month after month, year after year, they accomplished something amazing with long-term benefits to boot.

My lively friend Leona is another shining example of the benefits of swimming. She is 89 and loves the local indoor pool and the friends she meets there regularly. She's not there this week because she's on another trip with her attentive son, Dwight— her traveling companion. They travel often to fun places, but when she gets home, Leona's back at the pool with

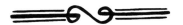

her lady friends.

Edna, 90, also enjoys going to the pool, and her favorite activity there is "water walking." She likes it because she can do it without "messing up her hair!"

Jim attributed his good health to doing daily calisthenics exercises for over fifty years. He started being intentional about it in his 40s and continued for half a century because he wanted to live a long, healthy life. He did. He lived—really lived—until he was 95. Jim's son-in-law told me, "Jim was a terrible example of aging. He didn't age."

Making a decision to do something good for yourself is one of the first steps toward living better longer. Being determined and dedicated to continue through the years is even more important.

Several months ago our daughter,

Christy, met a man named Bill who inspired her to start running. He said that he was 75 and had run over 60,000 miles. He bragged that he had been running every day for 28 years and 23 days. He was lean and fit and funny. Christy said something else also prompted her to get going. She was keeping Tucker, her friend's dog, and started taking him out for exercise each evening. She said she finally found a form of exercise she enjoyed and a time that fit her schedule, and that after two weeks it became a habit. Forming good habits, like adding something beneficial to our daily routine, takes TIME—in addition to our dedication and determination.

Vernon loves to golf. He's good at it because he's been working at it for many years. It is a healthy habit. Golf is a wonderful form of exercise because it is outdoors, usually in a pretty place; it provides camarade-

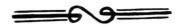

rie, companionship, and challenge. It keeps him and his golfing buddies engaged and active.

Gardening is another outdoor activity that provides pleasure, a sense of accomplishment, and meaningful movement. Being outside, digging in the dirt, and seeing something grow from seed to harvest, is rewarding.

Going to a gym or to the senior center to use the exercise equipment is another way some people stay in shape. I joined Curves and went for three hundred workouts...even got the t-shirt! The thirty-minute sessions using different types of machines provided a fun fitness regime. I'm still proud of my "300" shirt—my symbol of accomplishment and dedication. When we moved, I had to find other ways to keep moving. In keeping with the title of this book, I have to confess that dancing is my favorite form of exercise. I have been going to line dancing classes for ten years now. When we moved from one community to another, I was able to continue this group activity and make some new friends. I have found that it helps with flexibility, balance, and memory.

Two-stepping and waltzing around the living room by myself is also my idea of a good time. Dancing for exercise and singing along with whatever is on the Honky Tonk Tavern station is something I think is fun. I have probably danced enough steps to "Waltz across Texas" with Ernest Tubbs. As my friend Dr. William Purkey advises, I "dance like nobody's watching"—because nobody is.

Two friends told me about something they saw on *Dr. Oz* recently. They related that one of the guests on the TV show was sharing research about how dancing while singing along with the music is excellent brain exercise. Apparently, three different areas of the brain are engaged by this activity. The 21 year study they were referring to was from the New England Journal of Medicine and it showed that senior citizens who engaged in dancing frequently were less likely to suffer from dementia. Dancing that involves quick decisions challenges the mind and involves various brain functions all at once leading to increased mental acuity. The key is engaging in dancing frequently, though.[8]

In a 2014 edition of the *Blues Healthline* magazine, there was an article about exercise entitled, "One of the Best Things in Life is Free." The author says, "You won't pay a dime for these health benefits:

◇ Lowered blood pressure

◇ Reduced risk of cardiovascular disease and stroke

◇ Improved cholesterol levels

◇ Reduced risk for type 2 diabetes

◇ Reduced risk for certain cancers—including breast and colon

◇ Reduction of stress

◇ Reduction of anxiety and depression

◇ A good night's sleep

◇ Stronger muscles and bones to support healthy aging

◇ Enhanced psychological well-being

◇ More than three years added to your life."[9]

Find a form of exercise that you enjoy and stick with it long enough to make it a habit. Choose a regular time that fits into your daily schedule; put it on your calendar; program it as an app on your phone, and just do it! Get a move on! You're worth it!

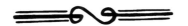

"Money can't buy the benefits of exercise, but they can be yours for free." ~Blues Healthline

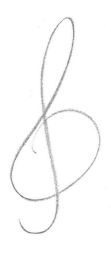

GuiDANCE:

What form of exercise could you commit to doing regularly?

chapter 17

She's a Mean Old Woman

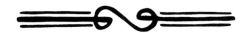

I bet the last thing someone would want to have said about them is, "She's a mean old woman." Her daughter-in-law said it, and her sister repeated it in agreement. It is sad that those who are closest are often the ones who receive the wrath. I won't say her name, but I feel I must

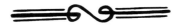

include this sad story because, in our quest to learn what to do, we can also learn what not to do.

Like a few others I've known, this lady has two separate personalities. Unfortunately, she shows her sweet self to strangers and saves her mean-spirited self for family. She complains bitterly about caregivers, berates her children and grandchildren, and despises her daughters-in-law. Nothing suits her.

Her last sister has resolved not to go see her anymore until she's dead. What can we learn from this sad state of affairs? There are those who are sweet in their senility. What makes the difference? I don't know. I'm not sure if she has Alzheimer's. She seemed sane when I saw her several months ago.

My observation is that this "mean old lady" (and a few others like her

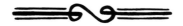

that I have known) alienated family and friends, and now, at the end of her life, finds herself alone, emotionally abandoned, and wondering why.

Lois, one of my wisest mentors, once told me that "whatever people are throughout their lives, they just become more that way as they age. If they are sweet, they get sweeter. If they are mean, they get meaner." These are not scientific, research-based observations, but they are her personal insights gleaned from 91 years of living.

I met a young woman recently who provides home health care and physical therapy for elderly patients. She said, "I've seen it all, and it has helped me to decide what sort of 'little old lady' I want to be." I think she's onto something. We do have a choice.

It has been said that our inevitable

trials and troubles can make us "bitter or better." I believe in the power of intentionality and that if we purpose in our hearts to age gracefully and sweetly, it will be so.

Several years ago I heard a story in a Sunday School class about an old woman who was no longer able to live alone and to take care of herself. Her family members were busy working and unable to safely care for her daily physical needs. They located a nursing home facility nearby and made preparations for the transition. As they were driving toward her new home, the mother said to her daughter, "I love it."

The daughter responded, "But Mom, you haven't even seen it yet."

"I know," she replied, "but that doesn't matter. I've already made up my mind. I love it." Imagine the load that was lifted from the daughter's

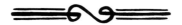

heavy heart when her mom expressed her intentions—her plan to be content in her new surroundings.

As Stephen Covey advised, we should "begin with the end in mind."[9] We can plan ahead. We can be intentional about what kind of spirit we choose to have and to project to the world. The good news is that we do not have to wait until we are old; we can start today.

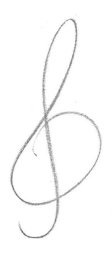

GuiDANCE:

Have you given conscious thought to kind of person you want to be?

chapter 18

The Chickens Do Come Home to Roost

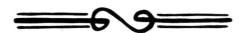

As I have interviewed and observed older people through the years, I have seen some sad things. My observations have been mostly positive, but I have found that there are some elderly men and women who get near the end of their lives and find themselves alone—estranged from family

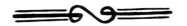

and with few friends. I've seen the forlorn faces of folks who sit day after day without visitors.

In some cases I have heard stories directly from the daughters of those who were basically abandoned at nursing homes. They told me that their mothers were always mean to them and that they felt no obligation to offer emotional or moral support or TLC (tender, loving care) in their final years of life.

The adult children of these women saw to it that basic physical needs were met, but they removed themselves from any care-giving role and kept their distance. After years of verbal abuse and, what they perceived and described as a lifetime of mistreatment, the daughters did what they felt they had to do for self-preservation. One of the lonely elderly women said to me, "I never thought they would treat me this way." She didn't know I

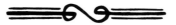

had heard the other side of the story.

I only saw the pious, sweet face she presented to the public, but I knew the other side existed. Again, what came to my mind was, "What goes around comes around..." Chances are good that your children will follow your example and treat you the way they saw you treat your parents.

I am not trying to judge either the mothers or the daughters. I'm just saying that it's a good idea to do your best to be a loving and kind parent. I heard someone jokingly say, "Be kind to your kids; they may choose your nursing home." That's not the main reason to be kind to your kids, but it might make a difference in the quality of your care.

Seeing these sad situations of estrangement made me appreciate, once again, the blessing of a lifetime of love from my precious mother and

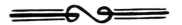

daddy. I am reminded of a statement from someone not as fortunate who said, "I wish I could have had a loving mother like Kate's." I know I was blessed, and I am very thankful.

I must also share some more positive observations of other daughters who were abandoned and/or abused by parents but who made a conscious decision to forgive their mothers and fathers later in life. The three who come to mind are strong, Christian women. Through their faith, they found a way to forgive. Each of these daughters did not continue the cycle of abuse and neglect. I observed that when their parents needed them, they intentionally chose to respond with love and forgiveness. These are happy, wonderful women who I admire greatly. Through their choice of love and grace, they were able to witness to their parents and to provide a good example for their children and

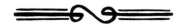

grandchildren.

Those adult children who chose not to forgive do not appear to be as happy as the others. Anger, bitterness, and unforgiveness are heavy loads to carry through life, and they take a costly toll.

If you are a mother or a father, I hope you will take inventory of how you are treating your children. Ephesians 6:4 states: "Do not provoke your children to anger, but bring them up in the discipline and instruction of the Lord." This verse can potentially help to improve all the days of your life.

The Bible also offers timeless advice on how children should treat their parents. The fifth commandment (Exodus 20:12) says, "Honor your father and your mother. Then you will live a long, full life in the land the LORD your God is giving you." It is repeated in Ephesians 6:2-3

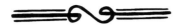

and states: "Honor your father and mother—*which is the first commandment with a promise*—that it may go well with you and that you may enjoy long life on the earth." NIV (Emphasis added.)

Ola Mae, one of the ladies I came to know, had a loving relationship with her 75-year-old daughter and all of her family. She was always teasing and reminding her children and grandchildren of the 5th commandment, and its promise. It was even mentioned at her funeral service. She must have been really good to her mother and father because she lived to be ninety-five years of age!

I remember years ago when my dear friend Lundee was lovingly caring for her aging mother. She said, "I will have no regrets." Her sincere words touched my heart, and I made a vow to follow her example.

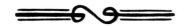

Whether we are talking about how we as parents treat our children or how we as children treat our parents, it seems that the trusty, time-tested, Golden Rule applies—"Do unto others as you would have them do unto you." Matthew 7:12.

The same principle can also be stated as: What goes around, comes around. In Galatians 6:7 we read, "You reap what you sow." Or, as Granny used to say, "The chickens do come home to roost."

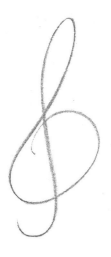

GuiDANCE:

What can you expect to reap from the relationship seeds you are sowing?

chapter *19*

What Goes Around Comes Around

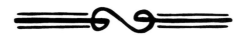

Ifirst met Gene when I would visit Mama at her assisted living apartment. Gene's wife was in the nursing home on the other side of the facility. Every day, on his way to see her, he would stroll through the dining room—standing straight and tall—greeting everyone with a warm smile

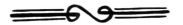

and a friendly hug. I noticed that the residents looked forward to seeing him.

Gene was the former chaplain for that home, and he knew the importance of his daily visits. I am certain that he saw it as a way to continue his ministry after his retirement. He faithfully followed this routine for nine years —until he was the one who needed someone to come and visit him.

When I first started interviewing folks for my pro-active aging project, I thought of Gene. I invited him over to our home, and Vernon listened as I interviewed him. We thoroughly enjoyed learning more about his interesting life.

As we were finishing with the final question, Vernon said, "He's your poster boy!" I agreed. It seemed as if Gene, at age 85, exemplified everything my research had revealed as important in a positive aging process. He had an amazing attitude, he exercised regularly, and he was a man of faith who studied his Bible religiously. His daily visits to see his wife and others that he met along the way gave his life meaning and purpose.

At the time of the interview, he was still writing a weekly column for the newspaper, and he had recently completed and published a book about his early life.

Several months after interviewing Gene, I was asked to speak about my research at the retirement home volunteer banquet. At the end of my talk, I called Gene up to the podium and presented him with the "Energizer Bunny Award" for being a shining example of a life well-lived. I bragged on how he kept going and going—always helping others.

One day, about a year later, I returned from an out-of-town trip, and I heard that Gene had moved from his home into assisted living. I hurried to go and check on him.

As I entered the building, I met a mutual friend and said, "I'm looking for Gene; I heard he was here."

"Oh, no," he lamented, "He's not here; he's on the other side," indicating the nursing home next door.

He continued, "I don't understand it; it's like he just gave up!"

"Oh my gosh. How can that be?" I asked, in dismay. I raced down the hall and dashed through the double doors that divided the two levels of care. When I stopped to ask someone where I could find Gene, they said something similar to the first person. They told me that he went on a trip to see his sister and that when he came back, he "just quit."

I located Gene's room. When I arrived, he was lying in the bed in a fetal position—looking frail and small. I frantically flipped on the light, and, without thinking, I blurted out, "Gene, what's going on?" I am sure I startled him out of a stupor. He seemed glad to see me, but there was a sadness about him that I had never seen before. We visited for a while, and I tried to assess the situation. Actually, it still remains a mystery to me today. He said several times, "I'm 87, going on 88," like that was long enough to live. I said, "Gene, you can't just QUIT! You can't just give up!" I was almost in tears as I added, "I gave you the Energizer Bunny Award! You have to keep on going...." I said sincerely, "I think you can live to be at least 96!"

That comment brought a smile to his face, and he did perk up a little. After I left his room, I went on a quest to bring Gene back to the "land of the

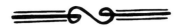

living." I called one of the elders of his church and asked him to get others to go and pray for Gene. I found the current chaplain and also asked for his prayers. I called one of the wonderful volunteers and asked him to go by regularly and encourage Gene. I talked to the nurses and aids and asked for their assistance in making a concerted effort to cheer him up. I prayed to know how to help this dear man who had helped so many others throughout his lifetime. I purchased flowers to brighten his room, made cheesy potato soup, and put his Energizer Bunny Award right where he could see it every day.

One day he mentioned that he liked cornbread and milk—buttermilk. I bought buttermilk, made some cornbread, and took it to him. That comfort food probably lifted his spirits more than anything else. He smiled and said, "I was 'raised up' on

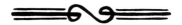

this stuff," and seemed to savor every bite.

The idea came to me to read his book to him. It was an autobiography called *The Pre-Atomic Age,*[11] and it told about his childhood and adolescence during the depression. It described how he survived after his plane was shot down during World War II. As I read what he had written, he would recall the stories and add other details of days gone by. We enjoyed our time together. It was a blessing that I will always remember. I was happy that he decided to stay a while—to linger longer...at least until we finished reading the book. I read slowly.

He rallied and seemed to be getting better for about six months, but he didn't make it to eight-eight. Each time I went to visit him, he would say, "Thank you for coming to see me."

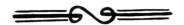

More than once I responded, "Do you know why I am here?"

When he would say no I would continue, "Because you're my friend, and because 'what goes around comes around.'" I would explain further, "for years I've been watching you come daily to visit Dorothy and the other residents. I've seen how you have blessed each of them. That's why I'm here for you now."

Every time we had that conversation, he would respond, "I don't remember that," and I would say, "Well, I do."

I still do....

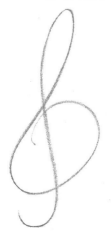

GuiDANCE:

Is there someone who needs to know you love, appreciate, and admire them?

chapter 20

To Find Out About the Road Ahead, Ask Those Who Have Traveled It

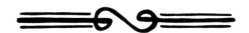

When I first began to think seriously about what we can do to age well—to live better longer—the idea came to me to talk to those who have traveled the road ahead to see what advice they would share. I decided to seek out those in my circle of influence who had done it right and

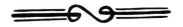

see what life lessons they had learned that would be beneficial. I also began to carefully observe family and friends and listen closely and thoughtfully to their stories. My parents and all my grandparents were gone by that time, but I reflected upon what I knew about my ancestors and determined to discern the legacy that they had left behind.

I have been blessed throughout my life by association with positive mentors. It was not a formal process of mentorship, but as I look back over my life, it is evident that special people have appeared in my life journey at just the right time—helping to influence and shape me.

My friend Dr. William Purkey says, "We are most influenced in life by the people we meet and the books we read." It has been ten years now since I first began my intentional journey to learn from lives well-lived. It is my goal, my ambition, my passion, and my purpose to put what I have learned into practice and to pass along ideas and inspiration to fellow travelers and to those coming behind me on the road of life.

In my quest to learn from those who have traveled the road before me, I've been intentional about asking for direction. This sage advice was given and received:

◇ Anonymous—"Pray to know which way to go; then, go as far as you can see on the horizon, and you can see farther."

◇ Stranger—"Figure out what you love to do, and find a way to get somebody to pay you to do it."

◇ Dean—"Take action. Start somewhere."

◇ Maggie—"Wear comfortable shoes."

◇ Dick—"Put one foot in front of the other."

- Mildred—"Take things in stride."
- Ruth—"Watch your weight."
- Earl—"Take your pills as prescribed."
- Joe —"Take your vitamins."
- Jack—"Exercise."
- Bennie—"Get good sleep."
- Willard—"Take life as it comes."
- Mary—"Go and do while you can."
- Betty Faye—"Be an intentionist."
- Emma Lee—"Be a *good-finder*. Look for the *good*."
- Lynn—"Do all you can do, then stand."
- Brian—"Be fully present. Wherever you are, be there."
- Clara—"Be happy."
- Harvey—"Hang around happy people."
- Helen—"Have friends of all ages."
- Lisa—"Be a good listener."
- Marquetta—"Count your blessings."

◇ Ronnie—"Hang on to hope."

◇ Betty S.—"Keep the faith."

◇ Ola Mae—"Honor your mother and father."

◇ Virginia—"Volunteer."

◇ Dorothy—"Tell them the value of 'replacement parts!'"

◇ Lois—"Stay active. Keep on keeping on."

◇ Marcella—"Don't let the things you can't do keep you from doing what you can."

◇ Clarice—"Read."

◇ Reid—"Stay interested in what's going on."

◇ Pat S.—"Keep singing!"

◇ Leola—"Keep dancing!"

◇ Evelyn O.—"Keep a positive attitude."

◇ Eula—"Always put God first."

◇ Craig—"Work hard to live a life of deep love."

◇ Dollie—"Be kind."

◇ Jerry—"Treat people the way you want to be treated."

◇ Pat B.—"Remember—relationships are *everything*!"

◇ Missy—"Forgive folks. Let it go."

◇ Pat H.—"Live in the present."

◇ Paul—"Finish strong. Stay the course. Stay faithful."

◇ Charles—"Keep your hands on the plow."

◇ Herb—"Never, ever, ever, quit!"

◇ Mackie—"Say your prayers."

◇ Roberta—"The most important thing is to love the Lord your God with all your heart and to love your neighbor as yourself."

◇ Grace—"Write this down and don't ever forget it: 'The Lord will take care of you.'"

"The wisdom of older per-sons needs to be shared in a

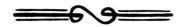

mentoring role with the next generations. We need to tell our own stories to younger generations so this valued wisdom will not be lost." ~Richard L. Morgan[12]

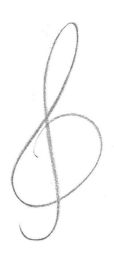

GuiDANCE:

What helpful advice have you been given?

What life lessons have you learned by observing those you have met on the road of life?

chapter *21*

The People We Meet

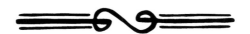

I met Marion at a campground in Colorado, and although it was only a brief encounter, we talked long enough for me to learn some life lessons. She was riding a bicycle when I first saw her, and she stopped to chat. She said she was 79 and would soon be 80.

She was friendly and welcoming, and we struck up a conversation. My friend Kathy knew Marion from the previous summer and had told me about her. They had often played cards together with some of the other camp ladies.

I was disappointed to hear that Marion and her husband would be leaving the next day. It was apparent that she was doing something right (to be riding a bike at almost 80 years of age), and I wanted to know what it was.

Marion seemed equally interested in learning about Kathy and me. She asked our names, where we were from, our birthdates, and said she was going to put that information in her journal. Kathy asked her to tell me about her volunteer work, so she related that she had served as a Pink Lady at the hospital for 35 years and now she visits regularly at the nursing home

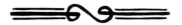

in her community. She told us about her family—her kids and grandkids.

Marion's positive, happy attitude was shining through everything she said. After she left, I assessed what I had seen and heard. What's Marion doing right to still be vibrant, joyful, and active after eight decades of life? She exercises; she plays games; she's interested in others; she has loving, caring connections with family and friends; she does meaningful volunteer work; she and her husband continue to "go and do," and, most of all, she does not have an *old* attitude. She is vitally alive and still enjoying life—still pedaling...still dancin'.

My chance meeting with Marion was enlightening. It was a reminder that everyone we meet has something to teach us. My dear friend Anita recently gave me a plaque with this old saying on it: "The Life You Live is the Lesson You Teach."[13] This anonymous

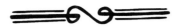

truth was first cited in print in 1918 and is still a popular quote that people hang on the walls of their homes and offices.

I want to share some of the specific things I have been taught by people I have met—some of those who have influenced my life. Some I only met in passing—like Marion, others I have known for over half a century. Most of them did not know I was paying attention and were not aware of the life lessons they were teaching me.

The two I want to tell you about first are prime examples related to the title of this book—two guys named Stan who were literally saved by dancing. Figuratively speaking, *Start Dancin' and Don't Stop* was meant to mean, live life with gusto, live life joyfully, live life fully for as long as possible. Actual dancing may or may not be part of the process. In the case of these two gentlemen, dancing was,

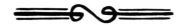

literally, a life saver.

Stan number one was married to Bessie for many years. They had no children and they had a very close relationship. After Bessie's long illness and eventual death, Stan seemed to die too. He set up a shrine to her in his living room with a poster-sized picture of his beloved as the centerpiece. Day after day he sat and stared at her picture, crying and pining away. After many months, some of her cousins intervened and invited Stan to come back to the land of the living.

They knew that Stan liked to dance and that he could really "cut a rug" in his younger years. He reluctantly accepted the invitation, and Bobby and Maureen finally got him to the dance floor of the senior center.

I saw him after he had been going there for a while, and he proudly said,

"I'm pretty popular down there." There were lots of lovely ladies who were happy to see Stan coming. One in particular caught his eye, and they began to dance together and keep company. Stan found a new lease on life. He and Rose eventually got married and continued to dance. The last time I saw them, they were waltzing around the dance floor at my Uncle Bennie's 85th birthday party.

The other Stan similarly lost his beloved wife, Mary, after many years of marriage. He was feeling down and seemed to have lost his zest for life. His daughter, Roxie, was getting worried about her usually joyful dad. One day at the senior meal site, he was asked to "jitterbug" for the group. Although he later said it was the longest dance of his life, the enthusiastic approval of his peers was a turning point for Stan. Loretta was there that day, and they discovered their mutual interest in dancing and began going often to towns nearby to dance. They enjoyed the companionship and became very close friends.

In both of these cases, dancing was the catalyst for a change of attitude. If you or someone you love and care about has lost their zest for life, dancing might be a good antidote. Finding something enjoyable to do with someone you love can be a cure for a lot of ails.

Last Saturday Vernon and I went to the local senior center for the weekly dance. The Old School Band was playing, and the room was full of fun, happy people who were having a really good time. They welcomed us, and we appreciated their warm reception. One gentleman who caught my eye was Prudie, age 95, who was on the floor for most every number. He told me that he started dancing when he was fifteen and had been "dancing ever since."

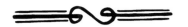

Vernon and I agreed that the people we met at the dance seemed to be the happiest group of people in town. The last time we saw that much excitement was back in the fall when our local football team won their 28th state championship. We want to be a part of the fun, festivities, and fellowship and plan to accept their friendly invitations to "Come back next week!"

"You never know how far-reaching your influence will be."

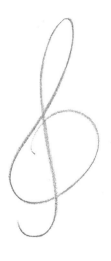

GuiDANCE:

What interesting people have you met while on your life journey?
Are there invitations you could accept that might help you live life more joyfully?

chapter 22

More People–My People

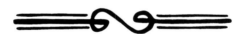

Vernon and I were driving down the highway and we were talking about our dear friend Ed who we called "Dado." He was part of our "framily" and he had just passed away at age 95. My mentor Betty Siegel taught me that "friends are the family that you choose for yourself," and the word "framily" perfectly describes our relationship with Dado. We were close friends for over forty years.

I asked, "What life lessons did you learn from Dado?"

Vernon said, "I don't know; what did he teach you?"

"Well, he taught me how to waltz and how to ride horses."

Vernon added, "He taught me how to skin an elk."

As we continued our conversation, we concluded that among many things Ed had taught us was the importance of having friends of all ages. We learned that you need friends older than you to share their wisdom and skills as well as friends younger than you who can come to visit you in old age. We discussed the value of making lots of special memories and sharing fun times that can be recalled

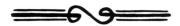

later in life. We often enjoyed visiting and laughing with Dado about old times together.

It is a reminder for all of us to be intentional about making happy memories that can be recalled and recounted as years go by. I love to take a lot of pictures and have found that precious old photos can prompt conversation and jar memories that may have been forgotten. Happy occasions can be re-lived and remembered more easily if there are pictures and videos taken and preserved.

However, there are everyday occurrences and conversations in life that are tucked away in our hearts and these treasures can also be brought to mind and privately savored and enjoyed again and again.

There are many people who have taught me much and I want to tell you more about some of them—spe-

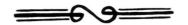

cial people I am blessed to know.

When I first began interviewing people for my project on pro-active aging, I thought of Reid and Marie, whom I knew from church.

They had invited Vernon and me over to their home for lunch, and we enjoyed their company and conversation. They showed us pictures and spoke proudly of their beautiful family—children, grandchildren, and great-grandchildren. They were a close and loving couple who created a good life and raised a wonderful family. They contributed much to the community and worked to make the world a better place. Their sweet spirits were what attracted us to them.

Marie is gone now and Reid has moved to a retirement home. He misses her much, but he continues to make the most of every day. He looks after the other residents, walks at least a mile daily, takes part in the activities offered, and always has a project going. At the age of 93, he is learning to play duplicate bridge.

He and his new friend David, another fine gentleman, have been working together to improve the memorial rose garden. The last time I went to see Reid, he was designing a mosaic tile plaque to place there in memory of Marie.

Reid and Marie are the kind of people I want to be like—good people. They have made a difference in my life and in the lives of many through their excellent examples of lives well lived.

Chuck is another one of my admired elders. This active nonagenarian (age 94) is someone we can all learn from. Chuck is the primary care-giver for his wife who he cares for in their home. He still goes to his office at the bank

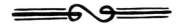

and maintains several investment accounts. He is an avid, outspoken supporter of Alabama football.

Most every Sunday he is in Sunday School—actively participating in the discussion. His mind is sharp and he also looks sharp in his black suit and tie.

Each week he faithfully serves as an usher during the church service. Chuck leads a purposeful life and is an inspiration to me and to many.

My Uncle Bennie is also an inspiration. He is now 87, going on 88. I love his optimistic attitude. As soon as he gets another candle on his cake, he is already counting on the next one. Aunt Mary says that although he has chronic pain, "he is like the Energizer Bunny who keeps going and going." He didn't let pain stop him from jumping out of an airplane when he was about 80. He does miss flying his

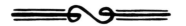

own plane and every day he wishes he could still do that.

He is very thoughtful about calling to check on my brothers and me, and he is always interested in what is going on in our lives. My brother Ronnie enjoys speaking to him in German. Uncle Bennie is intentional about keeping our family connection strong. He is now the patriarch of our family and is taking that role seriously. We are blessed to have his love and leadership.

Recently Vernon and I went to visit Mildred. When we got to her house, I didn't knock but just opened the door and yelled, "Yoo hoo," like Mama Dollie used to do. We all laughed and remembered days gone by when our families lived across the street from each other. There are millions of shared memories and "Yoo hoo" always conjures up some special ones. Mama and Daddy and Mildred and James were best friends for almost forty years. Daily conversations over coffee were the core of those relationships—the times when they shared their joys, their sorrows, and their secrets, and laughed and cried as they lived their closely connected lives. They traveled together to Branson, Nashville, Hawaii, and other vacation destinations. The four of them often played "42." The fellows went fishing and played golf; the gals shared recipes, homemaking tips, and weight loss efforts. When they reached retirement age, they all enjoyed fun and fellowship at the Senior Center.

The traditions they started continue because Mildred's son, Keith, and his wife, Ann, are our very close friends. We follow the friendship model of our parents as we stay closely connected through conversation over diet drinks, vacation travel in our 5th wheels, and playing rummy and mahjong. The fellows like to go hunting and fix things, and the gals like to play mahjong with girl friends and cook for one another. For several years Vernon and I lived down the street from them and that made it easier to get together. Since we have moved to another town, it takes more of an effort, but we are all intentional about keeping our friendship connection strong.

I give thanks for our five decades of friendship with Mildred and her precious family.

Another mentor of mine, whom I have known for over 50 years, is Lois. She is one of my "sheros" and someone I have always admired. I've known her since I was 12 and she is an amazing woman. She was my Sunday School teacher and youth group sponsor. She is 91 now and still has bright red hair and walks with a lively step. The last time I went to her home to

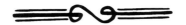

visit, she was playing solitaire while watching the news. "I can't sit still," she stated.

I call Lois my "Energizer Bunny" and consider her to be the epitome of a life well lived. She is full of perpetual energy that she has always directed toward helping others. She still gets more done than many half her age.

Recently she spear-headed the bi-annual rummage sale at the retirement home where she regularly volunteers. She is older than many of the residents, but she is still going strong.

Last Sunday she was honored at her local church with the "Living Legacy" award. Her leadership in the New Mexico United Methodist Women is unequaled, and she deserves recognition. No one will ever know all of the good she has done in her lifetime.

Her faith is strong, and she at-

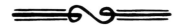

tributes her positive attitude to her close and personal relationship with the Lord. She is not a worrier and prays always for guiDANCE and assistance through daily life. She has blessed me through her example.

I am happy to tell you about these people, my people, that the Lord has blessed me with throughout my life. They have touched me; I have grown.

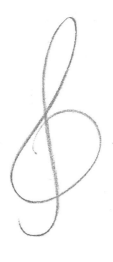

GuiDANCE:

Think about the men and women you know and have known who have influenced your life story.

chapter 23

The Books We Read

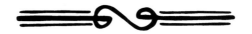

In 1988, after I spoke at the New Mexico State Toastmasters competition, a woman named Regina, whom I never saw before and have never seen again, appeared out of the crowd. She handed me a book and said, "I think you will like this." I thanked her, and she disappeared.

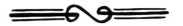

Apparently, something in my speech on "Intentional Invitational Living" struck a chord with her, and she was prompted to give me a present.

The unexpected gift she gave me has truly been a gift that keeps on giving. I have read and re-read that little book time and time again. The front cover is missing, the pages have fallen apart, and I have to keep it in a plastic baggie. The title of my little treasured treatise is *The Way Out*. The truth it contains has shaped my thinking and my life. As I mentioned earlier, William Purkey says: "We are most influenced in life by the people we meet and the books we read." Only the *Holy Bible* and *Inviting School Success* have influenced me as much. In this chapter and those that follow, I will share ideas that I have gleaned from this book and others like it.

The Way Out, written in the early 1900s by Joseph Benner under the pen name Anonymous, is not for everyone. In fact, through the years I have shared it with only a few people, and even the few I gave copies to didn't seem to get it. I'm not sure why it means so much to me and doesn't resonate with others. I recommend it to you with hope that you can find a copy and discover the truth it offers.

The message from the book that means the most to me is this: *"Whatever you think and hold in consciousness as being so, out manifests itself in your body or affairs."* It further states:

> You must train yourself to STAND GUARD CONTINUALLY AT THE DOOR OF YOUR MIND, AND TO LET IN NO THOUGHT OR FEELINGS THAT YOU DO NOT WANT TO OUTMANIFEST. Guard the door from every negative thought and feeling

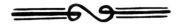

of whatsoever nature—from every thought that you know God would not have you think; from every doubt, fear, worry, anxiety or concern of any kind; from every tendency to criticize, judge or condemn anybody or anything or any condition; from self pity, jealousy, envy, irritation, unkindness, anger, hatred, etc. These will give you an idea of what are negative and unGodlike thoughts, and which must no longer have a part in your consciousness.[14]

The book also stresses "the importance of always being positive in your thinking, positive in your speaking, and positive in your doing." Although this is a tall order, I do believe we can choose our thoughts and that if we make a conscious effort to look on the bright side of life, we can be

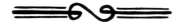

a *good-finder*. We will find what we focus on.

Words are powerful. The words we speak and the words we think determine our destiny. Positive thinking and positive speaking take an intentional effort, but we can do it. We are born with free will—the ability to choose our actions and attitudes. I call it "awillity." It takes our conscious awillity to pursue a positive path. None of us are perfect, but we can all do better when we try. If we make an intentional choice to be a certain way and ask our Heavenly Father to help us, we can change negative habits and live more positively all the days of our lives.

"Whatsoever things are true, whatsoever things are honest, whatsoever things are just, whatsoever things are pure,

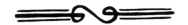

whatsoever things are of good report; if there be any virtue, and if there be any praise, think on these things." Philippians 4:8 KJV

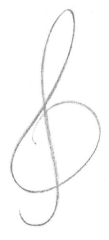

GuiDANCE:

Do you have the **awillity** to choose a positive way of life?

chapter 24

Change the Way You Think to Change the Way You Feel

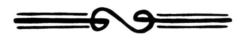

Another book that has influenced my life is *The Power of Positive Thinking*. When Dr. Norman Vincent Peale first wrote his classic best seller, there were naysayers and skeptics who doubted and debated his optimistic ideas. That book, written in 1952, has sold more than 7 million

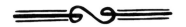

copies and has been translated into 15 languages. It struck a chord heard round the world—changing countless lives. Dr. Peale, the "Father of Positive Thinking," lived to be 95 years of age, and his wife Ruth, who also practiced a positive approach to life, lived to be 101. They both maintained their cheerful attitudes and modeled positive living until the end of their long lives. In the 60 plus years since this seminal book on positivity was published, research has validated Dr. Peale's hypothesis.[15]

I recently saw Dr. Richard Beeser on Good Morning America reporting that a "better attitude is correlated with a longer life." A study was conducted of 2,000 patients with heart disease, and they found that "thinking positively has positive benefits." Those who thought they could do more could do more, and it was concluded that your mind and thoughts play a significant role in how you do. Dr. Beeser stated that "upbeat attitudes are so powerful that they may become a part of health regime."

I am strongly suggesting that you intentionally make optimism and positive thinking and speaking a part of your health regime. If you really want to live better longer, start with your attitude. Your way of thinking not only improves your outlook on life, but also influences how long you actually live. In 2002, researchers at the Mayo Clinic in Rochester, Minnesota found that "optimistic people decreased their risk of early death by 50% compared with those who leaned more toward pessimism."[16]

In an article on longevity by Dr. Mark Stibich, he states:

"Research shows that how you perceive aging affects how long you will live. In a study of 660

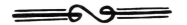

people, those with more positive perceptions of their own aging lived an average of 7.5 years longer. Adjusting your perception of aging while you are still young can have a tremendous effect on your life expectancy. No one knows for sure why a positive attitude seems to lead to a longer life, but research has shown that it does improve resiliency and help people to live better longer."[17]

I have some friends who "talk old" and seem to always view the aging process in a negative light. Although I make an intentional effort to encourage them not to say the "o" word, they persist. Hopefully, when they hear that seven-and-a-half years can be added to their lifespan by changing to a more positive perception of aging, they will change their 'tude.

My favorite Mary Englebreit greeting card contains this quote by D.F.E. Auber: "Aging seems to be the only available way to live a longer life." Since aging is inevitable, it seems that we should accept it, adjust our attitude about the process, and make conscious choices to control the things we can. Let's be like Edna. Her daughter-in-law bragged about how at eighty-something she was doing great. She said, "Edna has embraced this stage of life, and she's having a wonderful time."

An article called "The Upsides of Aging," by Monty Lyons, points out that "each decade, each age, has opportunities that weren't there before." He quotes from a book by Karl Pillemer, a gerontologist, who wrote *30 Lessons for Living: Tried and True Advice From the Wisest Americans*. As in all stages of life, attitude is key. "If your attitude is that you're still

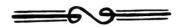

good, you still enjoy life, there's still purpose in your life, you'll do well."[18]

Embracing the aging process, viewing all of life as an adventure, and intentionally practicing positive thinking can help us live better longer. Fear not. Fear not.

In "Be Happy for Your Heart," an article by Linda Wasmer Andrews, she states: "An increasing body of scientific evidence suggests that happy feelings and an upbeat attitude are associated with better heart health and a longer life too." She suggests "tweaking your thinking," adding this: "People who are happy and optimistic look at problems as challenges and focus on finding solutions while unhappy, pessimistic people look at problems as permanent, and they throw in the towel right away."

She recommends counting your blessings as a way to improve your attitude. "Research has shown that people who express gratitude on a regular basis are more optimistic and healthier, on average, than those who don't."[19]

Grab a journal, a yellow note pad, or your computer and begin the daily habit of recording your blessings. Think of all the good things you have experienced in life. Give thanks for your abunDANCE. Just this simple step of focusing on the good things life offers can help to change your way of thinking and bring you joy.

Many years ago I presented a program called, "Be a Good-Finder." It was about purposefully focusing on the positive rather than the negative things in life. I used an illustration that has stuck with me for over forty years. I took a large white poster board and drew an oddly shaped dark spot in the center. I held it up and simply asked, "What do you see when

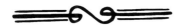

you look at this poster?" Everyone immediately began to examine the black shape to see what it looked like to them. "A dark cloud," "a worm," "a whale," they guessed—each one focusing on the small dark image on the large white board. After several minutes of examination, I stopped the discussion and asked them to look again at the whole poster. I pointed out that 99% of the poster was white, but that when I said, "What do you see?" everyone immediately honed in on the little dark spot.

Unfortunately, this is what often happens in life. Ninety-nine percent of things may be going well, but our first (and often our last) reaction is to focus on the negative, the dark side, the problems. I challenge you to be a "good-finder"—to shift your focus from what's wrong to what's right, to look for the positive rather than the negative, to change the way you

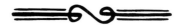

think, to change the way you feel, and you may just add 7.5 happy years to your life span.

"A cheerful heart is good medi-cine." Proverbs 17:22

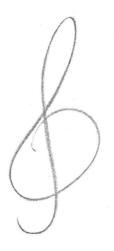

GuiDANCE:

Do you need to tweak your thinking?

chapter 25

You Can't Give Away What You Don't Have

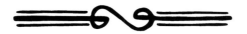

Nell was an inspiration to all who knew her. Every morning she would read the obituaries, and if her name was not among them, she joyfully bounced out of bed and made the most of her day. Another spunky lady who is 105 said, "I get up every morning and think about *living*." She

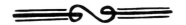

said she never thinks about dying.

Getting older is a blessing. It means you are still alive. Get up and get moving. Spread some cheer. Lift someone's load. Be a blessing to some-one else. One of my favorite lessons from the Bible is that "we are blessed to be a blessing." (Genesis 12:2) Each day pray for guidance to know who you can help.

My sweet sister-in-law Jeannine was a wonderful first grade teacher. Each morning as she turned on the light in her classroom, she said, "This is the day that the Lord has made. Let us rejoice and be glad in it." Quot-ing Scripture, like Psalm 118:24, is a wonderful way to start every day. Add it to your routine. I have placed those words, in large letters, on the wall of our home, and they serve as a daily reminder of where our Joy comes from. I want our home to be a "joy-ful refuge" and have been intentional about making it more inviting by putting the word JOY in every room. I also make every effort to put joy into our daily lives.

Think about what brings you joy. What makes you feel most alive? What makes your heart sing? Do more of it. Put it on your calendar.

If you are feeling as if you are out of joy, keep reading...

About twenty-five years ago, I found a book called *Out of Apples* by Lee Schnebly, and it offered some timeless ideas that have helped me and the countless others that I've shared the concept with. Lee was a young mother struggling with de-pression and discouragement. She went to a counselor who told her that her problem was that she was "out of apples." He suggested that she think of herself as an empty apple barrel. He observed that as a working wife

and mother and daughter and neighbor and friend that she had given and
given all her "apples" away and that
she had nothing left to give.

He wisely advised her to think of
those things that she enjoyed doing,
those things that brought joy to her
heart, and to intentionally do them.
"Whatever it is that is important to
you, you've got to see that you do it,
because that is how you get apples."[20]

You can't give away what you don't
have. If your emotional apple barrel
is barren, you need to replenish your
supply. Think of what brings you joy,
and do it soon—do it often.

When your barrel is full, you can
once again have apples to share with
others. You can more fully focus on
living joyfully all the days of your life.

**"Moreover, God has the power
to provide you with every gra-**

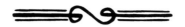

cious gift in abunDANCE so that always in every way you will have all you need yourselves and be able to provide abundantly for every good cause." Jeremiah 17:7-8 NLT

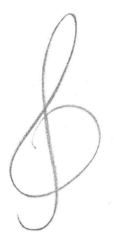

GuiDANCE:

Does your apple barrel need replenishing?

chapter 26

Get Your House in Order

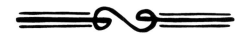

I just got a devastating phone call from my friend's daughter. She called with the news that her precious mom, Judith, had passed away very unexpectedly. She had just celebrated her 68th birthday with her family a few hours before.

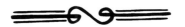

Last week, Carol, another sweet, sixty-something-year-old lady that I knew from Community Bible Study died just as suddenly. The week before I heard the sad news that Charles, a fellow "long-marcher" in the Alliance for Invitational Education, had passed away in his early sixties. These sudden losses give us reason to pause, reflect, and realize our mortality.

It happens. None of us have an assurance that we will be here tomorrow. That's why we have to take Pat's advice: "Live each day like it's your last."

You may follow all the advice given and ideas shared in this book and live to be 108, but you never know. There are no guarantees.

If we want to be among the "wellderly"[21]—those over the age of eighty who have no chronic diseases or ailments, there are steps we can take to improve the odds. The bottom line is that none of us knows how long we will have here on earth. I do not believe this is a negative thought, but rather, a positive reminder that each day is precious and that we should savor each hour, each encounter, and each blessing. As Warren says, "Every day is a blessing."

We can watch our weight, exercise, have a great attitude, and still get hit by a train or a drunk. So, it is a good idea to "get your house in order." No matter what your current age, there are certain things that can be done to bring you peace of mind and help your family in case something does happen unexpectedly.

A messy house can be a source of dismay and daily consternation. If your earthly home is in need of orderliness, Flylady.net is the answer. This system, created by Marla Cilley, aka Flylady, has helped millions of

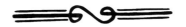

followers to take "baby steps" out of chaos and clutter into a more orderly and enjoyable existence. Through her book *Sink Reflections* and her daily email encouragement, Flylady can help you, literally, get your house in order. Her theory is that "you can do anything for fifteen minutes,"[22] and she will gently guide you toward tranquility in your home environment, fifteen minutes at a time.

Another helper, sent from Heaven in my opinion, is Dave Ramsey. He is an expert on money matters, and his TV and radio shows, CD series called *Financial Peace*, and his book *The Total Money Makeover*[23] have helped me and millions of others to get our financial affairs in order. Dave helps people work toward, and achieve, the goal of being debt free. Like Flylady, he urges people to take "baby steps" and he helps them to implement a plan for financial security. Start today by targeting and eliminating credit card debt. Live within your means. Get your financial house in order. Dave Ramsey can help.

Creating a simple A-Z filing system can eliminate much wasted time and frustration. Record all of your passwords in one place. Make a file listing all of your money matters. Account numbers, insurance policies, and vault combinations should all be recorded and placed where they can be located if needed. Tell at least one person where to find this information. The importance of making a properly executed will cannot be overstated. Get this done. At the same time, name a power of attorney, and let your final wishes be known.

Getting your house in order literally, financially, and figuratively is a good idea. Getting your spiritual house in order is also of utmost importance. Edna put it this way: "As a

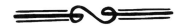

young person, I would play the piano in church. At an early time of life I thought, 'I want to be right with the Lord.' I really wanted to be right with Him." She wanted her spiritual house to be in order. At 90, she still keeps it that way by starting her day off "in the Word and in prayer." Is your spiritual house in order?

If you take inventory and find that some things need attention, it is not too late to get your house in order.

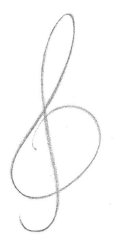

GuiDANCE:

Are there things you need to tend to, to get your house in order?

chapter 27

The Sun Still Shines Behind the Clouds

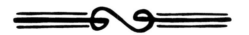

Sometimes life is hard. We have to face inevitable ups and downs that are just part of living. I have observed that those positive people of faith are better able to withstand the storms of life. One of my favorite quotes by Vivian Greene says: "Life is not about waiting for the storm to

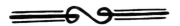

pass, it's about dancing in the rain."

Jackie, who has faced her share of tough times, told me, "God will give me what I need for this hard patch," indicating an optimistic view that "this too shall pass." I heard someone else who was not quite as positive, add to that old saying: "Yeah. It'll pass—like a pig through a python."

I know there are sad situations that seem like they will never end. It has been helpful for me to remember the phrase "the sun still shines behind the clouds." The storms will clear up. They are temporary, so keep on dancin'.

Years ago when I was feeling down about something that was troubling me, I went with Vernon to a meeting in San Diego. I decided to go over to the Convention Center to see what was happening. I followed a sea of people into the huge meeting room and found that Maya Angelou was about to speak. That seemingly serendipitous event had a profound effect on me. She told about her life and many challenges she had faced, and then, at the end of her talk, she sang a little song that continues to bless me to this day. She sang:

When it looked like the sun was never gonna shine anymore,

God put a rainbow in the clouds.

When it looked like the sun was never gonna shine anymore,

God put a rainbow in *my* clouds.

Maya Angelou was my rainbow that day. Although there were probably 10,000 people in the audience, I felt like she was singing that little song just for me. If you're going through a storm, a dark time, a cloudy day, or

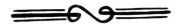

a hard patch, look for the rainbows. I believe God will send you a sign or someone to let you know He's there with you. We are not given a promise of life without sorrow or problems, but God did promise that He would be with us to help us weather the storm.

There's another song, sung by Rodney Atkins, that comes to my mind:

If you're going through hell,

Keep on going, don't slow down,

If you're scared don't show it,

You might get out 'fore the devil even knows you're there.

Keep on going. That's what I've learned from watching those who have weathered the storms of life. Persevere. Persevere. Take the next

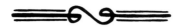

step. Put one foot in front of the other. Soldier on. Press on. Carry on. Keep the faith. Hang on to *hope*. Keep. Moving. Forward.

Some days are harder than others. I have some loved ones who have had to face horrific realities, and it seems they have had to make a conscious decision to keep on living. Although it was not easy, they had to make an intentional choice and *decide to move on*.

If you are at that point in life, you can do it.

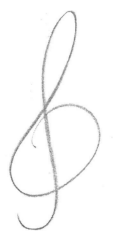

GuiDANCE:

Do you need to make an intentional decision to keep moving forward despite difficult circumstances?

chapter 28

That's Just Part of Life

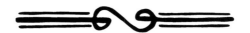

I've heard the expression, "That's just part of life" more than once through the years. After giving this some thought, it has come clear to me that having an attitude of acceptance of certain circumstances can make life easier.

Mildred said it to me after her husband fell and broke his hip and she sat by his side in the hospital for weeks. Ruth said it in reference to the loss of her husband after a long battle with cancer. Both of these strong women serve as examples of how to "carry on" after calamity. They were not angry or bitter, but they were resigned to the fact that "these things happen."

I am reminded of the Serenity Prayer by Reinhold Niebuhr:

God grant me the serenity to accept the things I cannot change, The courage to change the things I can, And the wisdom to know the difference.

Having the courage and the conviction to take action when we *can* make a difference is important. It is equally important to realize when we *can't* do anything about a situation. Praying for the ability and the wisdom

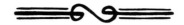

to *know* the difference can *make* a difference.

It is pointless to fret and worry over things that are out of our control. If we ask God for guidance to know what to do or not to do and then *listen*, serenity will follow. Peace will come.

When I asked Ruth if there was anything she would have done differently when looking back at her life, she said, "I don't think about that. There's nothing I can do about it now." This attitude of acceptance has helped her find happiness in her present stage of life.

My brother Ronnie often mentions the idea of "redrawing the map of the territory," which is a concept he learned in his graduate studies. An understanding of this idea can be beneficial as we deal with the inevitable challenges and changes that are

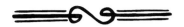

just part of life. This concept can be a helpful tool to carry with us on our journey.

"The map is not the territory," a phrase that was coined by Alfred Korzybski, "metaphorically illustrates the difference between belief and reality. Our perception of the world is being generated by our brains and can be considered as a 'map' of reality written in neural patterns. Reality exists outside our mind, but we can construct models of this 'territory' based on what we glimpse through our senses."[24] This is my interpretation of what I read: Our perceptions are not necessarily reality.

If you thought life would be a certain way, and it isn't; if your expectations have not panned out; if you can no longer do things you once enjoyed, it may be time to "redraw your map"—to rethink how you view a certain situation. *Changing your map may be as simple as changing your mind.* It can be a very positive way to deal with change.

This is my understanding of the process:

◇ Recognize that the map is not the territory.

◇ Be aware of your map of the territory

◇ Beware of false maps.

◇ Realize that maps change with time.

◇ Consider when it is time to revisit or redraw your map.

Recently a dear friend of mine, who was 93, said wistfully, "I wish I could still make the entire Thanksgiving meal for my family like I used to do." We talked about it for awhile, reminisced on how things used to be, and then found many current blessings. We drew this new "map of the territory." Maybe it is time for someone

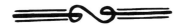

else to learn to make the dressing.

If a certain situation that is out of your control is causing you to fret or worry; if you think things should be a certain way and they are not; if your expectations have not materialized, try this. Rather than being disappointed, disillusioned, and downhearted, say to yourself, "That's just part of life, and there is nothing I can do about it," and redraw your map of the territory.

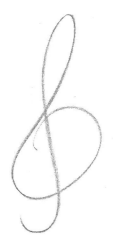

GuiDANCE:

Are there certain areas of your life where you need to redraw your map of the territory?

chapter 29

Live and Thrive and Until You Die

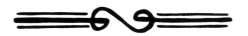

When I told my nursing educator friend, Cathy, about my interest in pro-active aging, she said, "You need to learn about compressed morbidity." It sounded like a morbid subject to me, but I decided to research it. Although it is a technical topic and not one we usually hear about, I

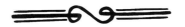

think it is something to which we all aspire. "Compression of morbidity is a term used to describe one of the goals of healthy aging and longevity...It is the goal of living disease and illness free for as long as possible."[25] To me, it means, "you live and then you die" —living as long as you are supposed to without prolonged illness and misery. If you and I want to be among the "wellderly," we can be intentional about choosing healthy lifestyles that can reduce, postpone, and prevent disease and serious medical maladies.

Another term Cathy taught me is "functional fitness" which refers to maintaining quality of life until you die. It means you can still get around and do what you need to do and want to do for as long as you live. Compressed morbidity and functional fitness make me think of the old guy who died on the golf course, or one I heard about the other day who fell over dead at 95—while dancing at his granddaughter's wedding. In both cases, people said, "That's the way he would have wanted to go," and they added, "I hope I can go that way too."

Just this morning, someone told me a story about how their beloved old family pet was "walking out the door to go pee, and he just died right there in the doorway." Mamaw, age 90, saw what happened and said, "that's how I want to go." Compressed morbidity—that's what it means to me. Live until you die.

The best example I know of this personally is Janie's mom, Jane. Janie had prepared a beautiful home in her backyard for her parents to live in when they retired and needed some assistance. They had a lovely home in Texas, but the time came when Janie felt that her mom and dad needed to be closer to her. She and her mom went to Boerne to pack things up and

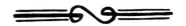

prepare for the move to New Mexico. After packing up a lifetime of memories, Jane sat down and said, "I wish I could just stay here until I died..." and then she did.

Compressed morbidity—you live and thrive until you die.

GuiDANCE:

Are you making healthy choices that will increase your chances of achieving compressed morbidity and functional fitness?

Will you be "wellderly"?

chapter *30*

Do Any Human Beings Ever Realize Life While They Live It

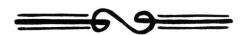

The phone rang and it was Marilyn. She asked, "Are you still working on your project about life?"

"Yes, it's a work in progress," I replied, eager to hear what she had to say. With Marilyn, you never knew what she would say next.

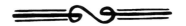

She continued, "Well, I've been thinking about it, and you need to tell them the importance of having a church family."

Marilyn had always been active in the Methodist Church—rarely missing a Sunday for over seventy years. She said, "I love my church family; they've been there for me all my life." She added, "I don't know what I would have done without them through the years—especially when my husband and son died."

We talked for a while, and then I thanked her for taking the time to call me with her ideas. When Marilyn called to share her thoughts, she had no idea that research had supported her observation that faith, prayer, and connection to a church community are correlated with fuller, happier, longer lives.[5] As I reflected on our conversation, I realized that Marilyn's reaction is what I hope will happen as you read this book. One of my main goals is for you to ponder what has been important in your life and to observe what has made a positive difference in the lives of others. The next step is to intentionally adopt or adapt those ideas, habits, and attitudes to create an optimal life.

I also hope you will share your observations and ideas about life and pro-active aging on the *Start Dancin' and Don't Stop* website—www. startdancin.com or send an email to kateasbill@gmail.com.

As I have talked to hundreds of people through the years, three re-curring themes have surfaced as most important—family, faith, and friends. When struggling with the loss of a loved one, many have said, "I don't know how anyone can make it through this without faith." The assurance of seeing their beloved parents, siblings, children, grandchildren,

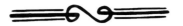

and friends again, in Heaven, carries them through that valley of life. It is comforting to have family and friends with us in our time of sorrow.

Family and friends also add to the joys of life. Holidays, birthdays, weddings, bar mitzvahs', quinceañeras, showers, and reunions can all be more joy-filled occasions because of precious time shared together in celebration. Just the daily living of life is more joyful when we are there for one another. There has never been a better time in history for staying connected to others. Instant communication is at our fingertips with our cell phones, computers, and iPads. One drawback with all this technology is that if you are constantly communicating with someone outside the room, opportunities for face-to-face conversation are lost. When gathering with family and friends for a meal, a party, a reunion, or for a few minutes, put the

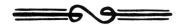

cell phone away and be fully present. Wherever you are, be there.

Perhaps it might help to look around the room and realize the importance of the moment—the significance of the *precious present*. Think of how you love those around you, what they mean to you, and seize the day. Take time to really talk to the people you are with, and learn what you can about their ideas, their dreams, and their lives. Share your own thoughts and aspirations. Be fully present.

I am reminded of a sad scene from *Our Town* by Thornton Wilder. Emily Gibbs, a young mother who dies in childbirth, asks to return to life for just one day. "Emily chooses to relive her twelfth birthday, but when she returns to earth, she discovers that people live their lives without appreciating or sharing the moments of living. They overlook the joy found in simple everyday activities."[26]

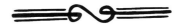

The poignant scene where Emily says, "Oh, Mama, just look at me one minute as though you really see me..." has a message for all of us. Although Emily's twelfth birthday was in 1899, the problem persists today.

She asks the Stage Manager, "Do any human beings ever realize life while they live it?"[27] That question can be a reminder to each of us to intentionally tune-in to life—to experience, appreciate, and relish everyday existence with family and friends.

Let's be like my friends Peggy and Charles who are intentional about celebrating life by often asking one another, "Isn't this a wonderful here and now?"

Realize life while you live it.

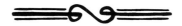

GuiDANCE:

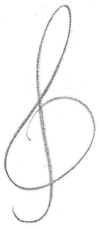

Are you being fully present to your loved ones, fully present to life as you live it?

Are you appreciating the "wonderful here and now?"

chapter 31

Love is What Keeps Me Going

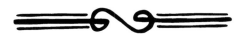

I gave a program about my research on what we can do to live better longer—how to thrive and not just survive. I loved it when several ladies added their thoughts on the subject. One of them said, "Read. Read as long as you can." Another shared what she had been told about the importance

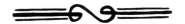

of accepting invitations. "If friends invite you to go and do things, you need to accept or they will quit asking."

Evie added, "Love is what keeps me going. It might be love for a person or even a pet." She's right. Well, they all are.

Love is a powerful motivator. I've seen several instances of the importance of beloved pets to people. One dear friend who lost her husband, the love of her life, told me how her sweet little dog helps her keep going. "Milo is my rock," she said. Dogs can be a source of unconditional love. Who else is going to jump up and down and wiggle their tail when you come home?

Getting a dog or a cat may help with loneliness, boredom, or self-absorption. It can also provide a source of exercise, but most of all, is the joy of companionship and love that animal

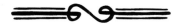

friends bring to life.

I've seen several examples of one person "holding on" to help someone they love. One precious friend who was diagnosed with cancer told his daughter, "I have to live long enough to take care of your mama." A son with a serious illness said to me, "I have to live long enough to take care of Mother." Both are continuing to live with purpose and devotion.

About twenty years ago, our family gathered to celebrate love as my nephew Wesley and his bride, Dana, were married. After the sweet ceremony, we were at the reception when we began talking about Mother and Daddy's upcoming anniversary, their 49th. Daddy had been diagnosed with cancer, but he was doing pretty well at that time.

I said, "Daddy, we want to have a 50th anniversary party for you and

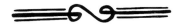

Mama next year and we really need you to be there."

He knew that was something special to her, and to me, so he said, "I think I can make it for a year."

I replied, "Well, we can't have that party without you, so we hope you'll be here—and if you can stay longer, that would be really good."

In November Daddy was told that his cancer was terminal. When he called to tell me the sad news, he said, "I'm gonna try to make it 'til March." He knew that party was important for a lot of reasons. He willed himself to live that long for the love of his wife and family.

Mother and Daddy married soon after he returned from World War II. They lived a happy life and raised three children (including me) in a peaceful Christian home.

I have two treasured letters that he wrote during his last year of life. The first one was written to our son, Corey, his grandson. He wrote: "When I got out of the army and came home, I was pretty well worn out and a nervous wreck. I met your grandmother, Dollie, who didn't have a middle name, so she gave herself one—"L," which means Love. She has more love in her heart than anyone I have ever known. She has been an inspiration to me to do better and be a better man. By her example she has had a great impact on all the people who know and come in contact with her."

Another letter written at the same time to my brothers and to me also talked about Mother's love. He wrote: "I have learned a lot from your mother about love. She has more love and compassion than anyone in the world. She has had a big influence in all our lives. There is not a thing I would change in our married life, as it has been a wonderful one. Not many rough spots at all. We had a few rough spots financially, but with the help of Sears Roebuck and Company, we made it through."

In January he became very ill and was hospitalized. We moved the party date to February and began to gather letters of love and appreciation from family and friends. Over 100 precious cards and letters filled with memories were compiled into a notebook.

On the day of the long-awaited 50th anniversary celebration, Vernon went to check Daddy out of the hospital for the day. He got dressed in his gold jacket and the gold and red tie that I bought for the occasion, and he looked so handsome. Mother looked beautiful in her pretty new red dress. It was a perfect day. All of our family and extended family were there. Although he was weak as the day started, you could see him gain strength as he and Mother were surrounded by their loved ones—kids, grandkids, siblings and spouses, cousins, nieces, nephews, special close friends, and even one of Daddy's aunts. Many came over 500 miles to help celebrate Dollie and John's fifty years together. Some of their childhood friends made the long trip from Texas to New Mexico to show their love and support. The pictures and our memories from that day capture a highlight in our family history. Love filled the room. It was almost tangible.

Daddy called me the next day from the hospital and he thanked me for the party and, especially, for the book of loving letters. He said: "We read those letters and we laughed and we cried, and we laughed until we cried." I still have the letters and it's amazing to see the little things

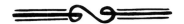

people remembered as important in their relationships with Mother and Daddy.

After the party Daddy lived five more weeks, and he did make it 'til March.

My mother and daddy, Dollie and John, didn't tell me how to live; they quietly showed me how to live. They lived and let me watch. They taught me much about life and especially about unconditional love.

I've seen several instances of long-married couples who passed away within hours, days, or weeks of one another. My great-grandparents, Mommie and Paw, are an example of that. She died, and nine days later he did too. Earlier, when they celebrated their 65th wedding anniversary, some-one asked, "Mommie, how did you and Paw stay together so long?"

She said, "Well, honey, it wasn't

easy. At first we were like a couple of young mules harnessed together—each wanting to go our own separate way. After a while we figured out that it works a lot better if you both just pull together."

She wanted us to know that marriage isn't always easy and that you have to make an effort to make it work. Prudie, 96, told me something that seems to fit this topic.

He was telling me about dancing with a lady-friend and he said, "We were dancing and it wasn't working very well until we figured out that she was doing a two-step and I was doing a waltz." That could be the case in other rocky relationships.

I think the sweetest and simplest thought on lasting love and peaceful existence is what Sandra said, "We're just nice to each other."

How hard is that?

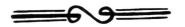

"And now these three remain: faith, hope and love. But the greatest of these is love." 1 Corinthians 13:13

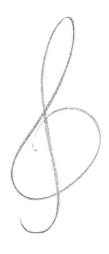

GuiDANCE:

Do you demonstrate and express your love for family and friends?

Is there someone who needs to hear you say, "I love you?"

chapter 32

In The Final Analysis

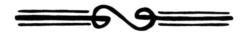

As I am nearing completion of this book, I want to come to some final conclusions about what I have learned through the process. Dr. Purkey taught me that "the process is as important as the product," and that is certainly the case in my ten year process of researching and writ-

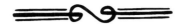

ing *Start Dancin' and Don't Stop!*

I called my friend Suzy who has worked at a funeral home for many years. I was curious to hear her observations about what is important in the final analysis of life. She quickly responded, "It's all about the close relationships that you've had, and did you leave the world a better place? It's not about the education. It's not about the money. It's not about possessions."

She recalled one dad who died after a long life. He was "Dr. So and So" and had a long list of accomplishments and publications, but when she asked his adult children to share something personal about their father, they couldn't. They said, "We never knew him."

Suzy continued, "This sums it up: It's the little things that matter most."

Vernon, who has lived with me

through this quest, also summed it up well. I asked him, "In the final analysis, what's important in life? What helps people live better longer?"

He said simply: "Family, faith, and friends." I was not surprised. Eleven years ago when he ran for the New Mexico State Senate, that was his platform. But family, faith, friends (and freedom) was not just a campaign slogan. It is a way of life—his way of life.

When I think about our parents and other lives well-lived, I recall that their lives also revolved around those three things.

Ross, one of my high school classmates, recently passed away very unexpectedly. I had been communicating with him through email and had enjoyed reminiscing about an old photo from our senior year. That picture served as a reminder of a fun, carefree day shared with friends in the mountains at Cloudcroft, NM. It will soon be fifty years since our graduation from Jal High School and an invitation to our "Blue and Golden Anniversary" party prompted our conversation. The party is going to be held at The Lodge in Cloudcroft—the same place where that old photo was taken. Although Ross said he would not be able to attend because of some health problems, I had no idea he would soon be gone.

After his death, I re-read our correspondence, and something he said had new significance. We were remembering old friends and he named several who were part of his fondest memories from growing up. Most were kids he went to church with and attended youth activities with during our childhood and adolescence. All those he named were, and still are, significant in my life as well. He said,

"I wish I could just spend a day with Keith and another with Paula." I knew what he meant. Keith, and his sister Paula, are also part of my treasured memories and my life-long friends. I'm not sure if Ross knew that his days were numbered when he said that, but I think he did, and seeing precious old friends once again was what was on his mind.

Think about what old friends you would like to spend a day with, and if that's not possible, give them a call or write them a letter.

When I called Aunt Doris to hear about her appointment with the oncologist, I wasn't prepared to hear what she had to say. She sadly shared that she had lung cancer that had spread and that the doctor said that she had only two to six weeks to live. She was just 83 and had always been so full of life that I could not imagine that she would soon be dead. Her

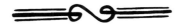

mother, Maw, had lived to be 96 and I had hoped Aunt Doris would too.

I called my brother Perry to tell him the prognosis and we decided he would fly down to get me, and that we would go see her. He told our Uncle Bennie that we were coming and Bennie called his sister to let her know. When Aunt Doris heard that we were flying from New Mexico to see her in Texas, she said, "Why didn't they just wait?"

"Wait for what?" Bennie asked.

"Till I died," she replied.

"Because they want to see you before you go," he said.

He was right. We did want to see her one more time and show our love and concern for her and the rest of the family. We wanted to let her know how special she was to us. We were able to express our love for her and to recall fond memories of many good times that we had shared.

We went back again three weeks later for her funeral. When I think about her last 21 days of life, I think of love in action. Her family members all showed up to minister to her in a variety of ways—each one personally demonstrating their care and love in a different manner.

Her grandson-in-law, Rob, was like an angel—caring for her needs. Soon after her diagnosis, Rob said, "Doie, you and Papa have traveled to many beautiful places; is there any place you'd like to go again?"

She smiled sweetly and said, "I'd just like to go to church."

Although she did not get to go to church again, church came to her. Her church family prayed for her comfort and brought food. Lots of food. Many who loved her came to visit.

I was honored when Uncle Gene said, "I want Kate to do the eulogy." Aunt Doris had always been very dear to me, and I was blessed to be able to share some special memories of a life well-lived. Like her mother, Maw, and her sister, Dollie, she left us with a legacy of *love*—love for the Lord, love for others, and love for life. The unwavering love that she had always given out came back to her in her final days.

As I talked to those who knew her best, we told stories of great times together and laughed at her antics. She was known for her wonderful sense of humor and spirit of *fun*.

A favorite memory of everyone was how she always led the Muldoon Fourth of July parade—wearing red, white, and blue and a crown and waving from her throne—a recliner attached with baling wire to a front end loader. She was in her element—

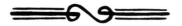

bringing smiles to her "subjects" who lined the road to see her.

When preparing remarks for her celebration of life, it came clear to me again that *family, faith, friends*, and the *making and remembering of precious memories* are what matter most.

In the final analysis, I believe these essential elements are what make life worth living and help us to live better longer. They will not only add years to your life, but life to your years. Be intentional about focusing on these priorities.

In addition to those vital elements for a joy-filled life, also be *intentional* about these things:

◇ Be positive.

◇ Take care of yourself.

◇ Nurture relationships.

◇ Go and do.

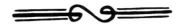

◇ Take pictures to help preserve memories.

◇ Give thanks for your abunDANCE.

◇ Pray for guiDANCE.

◇ Have a wonderful life.

◇ Don't quit.

◇ Keep on DANCIN'...

◇ Finish strong.

AND, if you want to live forever, remember John 3:16

> **"For God so loved the world that He gave his one and only Son, that whoever believes in him shall not perish but have *eternal* life." (emphasis added)**

I hope that as you read *Start Dancin'* *and Don't Stop* you were reminded of people in your circle of friends and family who knew the secrets to living well longer. I would love for you to share their wisdom with me and with my readers.

To share their stories or other snippets of wisdom you have learned along the way, just go to my website www.startdancin.com or send an email to kateasbill@gmail.com to tell me about those special people in your life and what you have learned from them.

Footnotes

1 Purkey, William Watson., and John M. Novak. "The Inviting Approach." *Inviting School Success: A Self-concept Approach to Teaching, Learning, and Democratic Practice*. Belmont, CA: Wadsworth Pub., 1996. 50-55. Print.

2 "How to Live a Longer, Healthier Life." *Duke Medicine Health News* 14 G (2014): 3. Print.

3 "Life-Altering Lessons." *Blues Healthline* Issue 1 (2009): 8-9. Print.

4 Jaret, Peter. "Eight Facts About Diabetes That Could Save Your Life." *AARP Bulletin* 55.8 (2014): 10-11. Print.

5 Murawski, John. "Duke's Harold Koenig Completing Major Study on Faith and Healing."*NewsObserver.com*. N.p., 2 Feb. 2014. Web. 30 Dec. 2014.

6 Feingold, Ronald S. "Shaping Up." *Live Longer, Live Better: Adding Years to Your Life and Life to Your Years*. Pleasantville, NY: Reader's Digest Association, 1995. 92. Print.

7 Feingold, Ronald S. "Shaping Up." *Live Longer, Live Better: Adding Years to Your Life and Life to Your Years*. Pleasantville, NY: Reader's Digest Association, 1995. 124. Print.

8 Verghese, Joe. et al. "Leisure Activities and the Risk of Dementia in the Elderly." *The New England Journal of Medicine* June 2003.

9 "One of the Best Things in Life Is Free." *Blues Healthline* Issue 4 (2014): 16. Print.

10 Covey, Steven. "Habit 2: Begin with the End in Mind." *The Seven Habits of Highly Effective People*. Provo, UT: Covey Leadership Center, 1996. 50-77. Print.

11 Fooks, Leslie Eugene. *The Pre-Atomic Age*. Victoria, B.C.: Trafford, 2006. Print.

12 Morgan, Richard Lyon. *Remembering Your Story: Creating Your Own Spiritual Biography Revised Edition*. Nashville: Upper Room, 2002. Print.

13 "The Big Apple: "The Life You Live Is the Lesson You

Teach".” *The Big Apple: "The Life You Live Is the Lesson You Teach”.* N.p., 18 Dec. 2012. Web. 18 June 2015.

14 Benner, Joseph. "The Law." *The Way Out.* Marina Del Rey, CA: DeVorss, 1971. 12, 17+. Print.

15 Peale, Norman Vincent. *The Power of Positive Thinking.* New York: Prentice-Hall, 1952. Print.

16 "15 Ways to Live Longer." Forbes.com, n.d. Web. 26 Oct. 2006.

17 Stibich, Mark, Ph.D. "Think Positive About Aging and Live Longer." (n.d.): 1-2. *About.com.* 26 Apr. 2009. Web. 13 Nov. 2010.

18 Lyons, Molly. "The Upsides of Aging." *USAWEEKEND* 4 Nov. 2011: 4. Print.

19 Andrews, Linda Wasmer. "Be Happy for Your Heart." *American Profile* 24 Feb. 2008: 4. Print.

20 Schnebly, Lee. "Introduction." *Out of Apples?: Understanding Personal Relationships.* Tucson, AZ: Fisher, 1988. 1. Print.

21 Hall, Stephen S. "New Clues to a Longer Life." *National Geographic* 223.5 (2013): 28-49. Print.

22 Cilley, Marla. *Sink Reflections.* New York: Bantam, 2002. Print.2

23 Ramsey, Dave. *The Total Money Makeover: A Proven Plan for Financial Fitness.* S.l.: Thomas Nelson, 2007. Print.

24 "The Map Is Not the Territory." - *Lesswrongwiki.* N.p., 3 Dec. 2012. Web. 18 June 2015. <http://wiki.lesswrong.com/wiki/The_map_is_not_the_territory>.

25 Stibich, Mark. "Compression of Morbidity - Reducing Age-Related Suffering." *About.com.* N.p., 29 Oct. 2013. Web. 18 June 2015.

26 Snodgrass, Mary Ellen., and Thornton Niven. Wilder. "Brief Plot Synopsis." *Cliff Notes on Wilder's Our Town.* Lincoln, NE: Cliff Notes, 1990. 12. Print.

27 Wilder, Thornton. "Act III." *Our Town A Play in Three Acts.* New York, NY: HarperCollins, 2003. 107-08. Print.